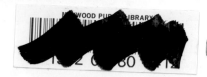 

MAYWOOD PUBLIC LIBRARY

W9-BUB-854

DATE

MAYWOOD PUBLIC LIBRARY
121 SOUTH 5th AVE.
MAYWOOD, ILL. 60153

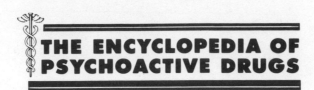

THE ENCYCLOPEDIA OF PSYCHOACTIVE DRUGS

SERIES 1

The Addictive Personality
Alcohol and Alcoholism
Alcohol Customs and Rituals
Alcohol Teenage Drinking
Amphetamines Danger in the Fast Lane
Barbiturates Sleeping Potion or Intoxicant?
Caffeine The Most Popular Stimulant
Cocaine A New Epidemic
Escape from Anxiety and Stress
Flowering Plants Magic in Bloom
Getting Help Treatments for Drug Abuse
Heroin The Street Narcotic
Inhalants The Toxic Fumes

LSD Visions or Nightmares?
Marijuana Its Effects on Mind & Body
Methadone Treatment for Addiction
Mushrooms Psychedelic Fungi
Nicotine An Old-Fashioned Addiction
Over-The-Counter Drugs Harmless or Hazardous?
PCP The Dangerous Angel
Prescription Narcotics The Addictive Painkillers
Quaaludes The Quest for Oblivion
Teenage Depression and Drugs
Treating Mental Illness
Valium The Tranquil Trap

SERIES 2

Bad Trips
Brain Function
Case Histories
Celebrity Drug Use
Designer Drugs
The Downside of Drugs
Drinking, Driving, and Drugs
Drugs and Civilization
Drugs and Crime
Drugs and Diet
Drugs and Disease
Drugs and Emotion
Drugs and Pain
Drugs and Perception
Drugs and Pregnancy
Drugs and Sexual Behavior

Drugs and Sleep
Drugs and Sports
Drugs and the Arts
Drugs and the Brain
Drugs and the Family
Drugs and the Law
Drugs and Women
Drugs of the Future
Drugs Through the Ages
Drug Use Around the World
Legalization A Debate
Mental Disturbances
Nutrition and the Brain
The Origins and Sources of Drugs
Substance Abuse Prevention and Cures
Who Uses Drugs?

NUTRITION
&
THE BRAIN

GENERAL EDITOR
Professor Solomon H. Snyder, M.D.
*Distinguished Service Professor of
Neuroscience, Pharmacology, and Psychiatry at
The Johns Hopkins University School of Medicine*

•

ASSOCIATE EDITOR
Professor Barry L. Jacobs, Ph.D.
*Program in Neuroscience, Department of Psychology,
Princeton University*

•

SENIOR EDITORIAL CONSULTANT
Joann Rodgers
*Deputy Director, Office of Public Affairs at
The Johns Hopkins Medical Institutions*

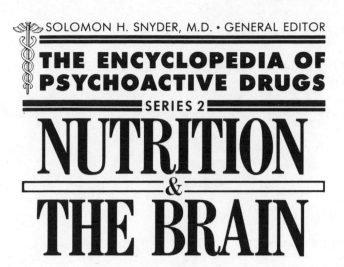

SOLOMON H. SNYDER, M.D. • GENERAL EDITOR

THE ENCYCLOPEDIA OF PSYCHOACTIVE DRUGS

SERIES 2

NUTRITION & THE BRAIN

EDWARD EDELSON

CHELSEA HOUSE PUBLISHERS

NEW YORK • NEW HAVEN • PHILADELPHIA

EDITOR-IN-CHIEF: Nancy Toff
EXECUTIVE EDITOR: Remmel T. Nunn
MANAGING EDITOR: Karyn Gullen Browne
COPY CHIEF: Juliann Barbato
PICTURE EDITOR: Adrian Allen
ART DIRECTOR: Giannella Garrett
MANUFACTURING MANAGER: Gerald Levine

Staff for NUTRITION AND THE BRAIN

SENIOR EDITOR: Jane Larkin Crain
ASSOCIATE EDITOR: Paula Edelson
ASSISTANT EDITOR: Michele A. Merens
EDITORIAL ASSISTANT: Laura-Ann Dolce
COPYEDITORS: Sean Dolan, Gillian Bucky, Ellen Scordato, Michael A. Goodman
ASSOCIATE PICTURE EDITOR: Juliette Dickstein
PICTURE RESEARCHERS: Jean Cantu, Debra P. Hershkowitz
DESIGNER: Victoria Tomaselli
PRODUCTION COORDINATOR: Laura McCormick
COVER ILLUSTRATION: Amanda Wilson

CREATIVE DIRECTOR: Harold Steinberg

Copyright © 1988 by Chelsea House Publishers, a division of Main Line Book Co. All rights reserved. Printed and bound in the United States of America.

First Printing

1 3 5 7 9 8 6 4 2

Library of Congress Cataloging in Publication Data

Edelson, Edward, 1932–
  Nutrition and the brain.
  (The Encyclopedia of psychoactive drugs. Series 2)
  Bibliography: p.
  Includes index.
  1. Brain—Juvenile literature. 2. Nutrition—Juvenile
literature. [1. Brain. 2. Nutrition] I. Title. II. Series.
QP376.E33 1987 612'.822   87–7999

ISBN 1-55546-210-3

CONTENTS

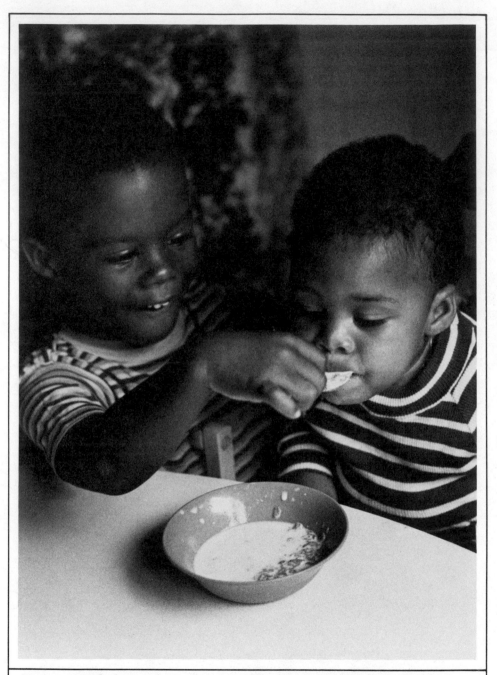

Young people have always been taught that eating the right foods can make them physically strong and healthy. Interestingly, some startling scientific findings are beginning to reveal a connection between nutrition and mental health as well.

FOREWORD

In the Mainstream
of American Life

One of the legacies of the social upheaval of the 1960s is that psychoactive drugs have become part of the mainstream of American life. Schools, homes, and communities cannot be "drug proofed." There is a demand for drugs — and the supply is plentiful. Social norms have changed and drugs are not only available—they are everywhere.

But where efforts to curtail the supply of drugs and outlaw their use have had tragically limited effects on demand, it may be that education has begun to stem the rising tide of drug abuse among young people and adults alike.

Over the past 25 years, as drugs have become an increasingly routine facet of contemporary life, a great many teenagers have adopted the notion that drug taking was somehow a right or a privilege or a necessity. They have done so, however, without understanding the consequences of drug use during the crucial years of adolescence.

The teenage years are few in the total life cycle, but critical in the maturation process. During these years adolescents face the difficult tasks of discovering their identity, clarifying their sexual roles, asserting their independence, learning to cope with authority, and searching for goals that will give their lives meaning.

Drugs rob adolescents of precious time, stamina, and health. They interrupt critical learning processes, sometimes forever. Teenagers who use drugs are likely to withdraw increasingly into themselves, to "cop out" at just the time when they most need to reach out and experience the world.

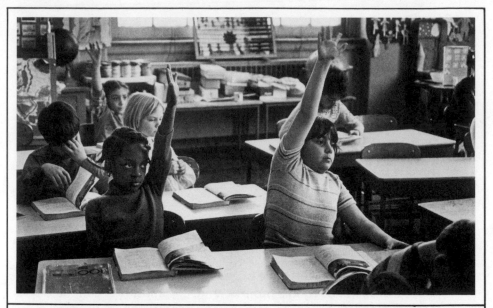

Education is a vital weapon in the war against substance abuse. Classroom discussions teach students that the brain regulates mood and perception and that these functions can be altered by drugs.

Fortunately, as a recent Gallup poll shows, young people are beginning to realize this, too. They themselves label drugs their most important problem. In the last few years, moreover, the climate of tolerance and ignorance surrounding drugs has been changing.

Adolescents as well as adults are becoming aware of mounting evidence that every race, ethnic group, and class is vulnerable to drug dependency.

Recent publicity about the cost and failure of drug rehabilitation efforts; dangerous drug use among pilots, air traffic controllers, star athletes, and Hollywood celebrities; and drug-related accidents, suicides, and violent crime have focused the public's attention on the need to wage an all-out war on drug abuse before it seriously undermines the fabric of society itself.

The anti-drug message is getting stronger and there is evidence that the message is beginning to get through to adults and teenagers alike.

The Encyclopedia of Psychoactive Drugs hopes to play a part in the national campaign now underway to educate young people about drugs. Series 1 provides clear and comprehensive discussions of common psychoactive substances, outlines their psychological and physiological effects on the mind and body, explains how they "hook" the user, and separates fact from myth in the complex issue of drug abuse.

Whereas Series 1 focuses on specific drugs, such as nicotine or cocaine, Series 2 confronts a broad range of both social and physiological phenomena. Each volume addresses the ramifications of drug use and abuse on some aspect of human experience: social, familial, cultural, historical, and physical. Separate volumes explore questions about the effects of drugs on brain chemistry and unborn children; the use and abuse of painkillers; the relationship between drugs and sexual behavior, sports, and the arts; drugs and disease; the role of drugs in history; and the sophisticated drugs now being developed in the laboratory that will profoundly change the future.

Each book in the series is fully illustrated and is tailored to the needs and interests of young readers. The more adolescents know about drugs and their role in society, the less likely they are to misuse them.

Joann Rodgers
Senior Editorial Consultant

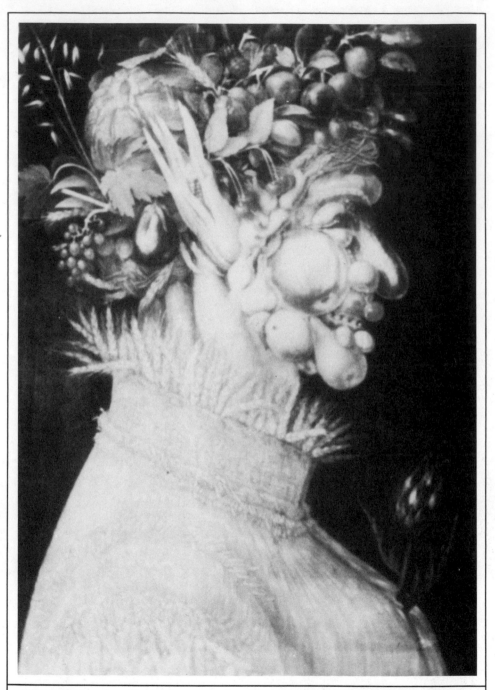

This painting by the 16th-century artist Arcimboldo fancifully depicts the old saying "You are what you eat." In fact, what you eat can produce changes in brain chemistry in a matter of minutes.

INTRODUCTION

The Gift of Wizardry
Use and Abuse

JACK H. MENDELSON, M.D.
NANCY K. MELLO, Ph.D.

Alcohol and Drug Abuse Research Center
Harvard Medical School—McLean Hospital

Dorothy to the Wizard:

"I think you are a very bad man," said Dorothy.
"Oh no, my dear; I'm really a very good man; but I'm a very bad Wizard."
—from THE WIZARD OF OZ

Man is endowed with the gift of wizardry, a talent for discovery and invention. The discovery and invention of substances that change the way we feel and behave are among man's special accomplishments, and, like so many other products of our wizardry, these substances have the capacity to harm as well as to help. Psychoactive drugs can cause profound changes in the chemistry of the brain and other vital organs, and although their legitimate use can relieve pain and cure disease, their abuse leads in a tragic number of cases to destruction.

Consider alcohol — available to all and yet regarded with intense ambivalence from biblical times to the present day. The use of alcoholic beverages dates back to our earliest ancestors. Alcohol use and misuse became associated with the worship of gods and demons. One of the most powerful Greek gods was Dionysus, lord of fruitfulness and god of wine. The Romans adopted Dionysus but changed his name to Bacchus. Festivals and holidays associated with Bacchus celebrated the harvest and the origins of life. Time has blurred the images of the Bacchanalian festival, but the theme of drunkenness as a major part of celebration has survived the pagan gods and remains a familiar part of modern society. The term "Bacchanalian Festival" conveys a more appealing image than "drunken orgy" or "pot party," but whatever the label, drinking alcohol is a form of drug use that results in addiction for millions.

The fact that many millions of other people can use alcohol in moderation does not mitigate the toll this drug takes on society as a whole. According to reliable estimates, one out of every ten Americans develops a serious alcohol-related problem sometime in his or her lifetime. In addition, automobile accidents caused by drunken drivers claim the lives of tens of thousands every year. Many of the victims are gifted young people, just starting out in adult life. Hospital emergency rooms abound with patients seeking help for alcohol-related injuries.

Who is to blame? Can we blame the many manufacturers who produce such an amazing variety of alcoholic beverages? Should we blame the educators who fail to explain the perils of intoxication, or so exaggerate the dangers of drinking that no one could possibly believe them? Are friends to blame — those peers who urge others to "drink more and faster," or the macho types who stress the importance of being able to "hold your liquor"? Casting blame, however, is hardly constructive, and pointing the finger is a fruitless way to deal with the problem. Alcoholism and drug abuse have few culprits but many victims. Accountability begins with each of us, every time we choose to use or misuse an intoxicating substance.

It is ironic that some of man's earliest medicines, derived from natural plant products, are used today to poison and to intoxicate. Relief from pain and suffering is one of society's many continuing goals. Over 3,000 years ago, the Therapeutic Papyrus of Thebes, one of our earliest written records, gave instructions for the use of opium in the treatment of pain. Opium, in the form of its major derivative, morphine, and similar compounds, such as heroin, have also been used by many to induce changes in mood and feeling. Another example of man's misuse of a natural substance is the coca leaf, which for centuries was used by the Indians of Peru to reduce fatigue and hunger. Its modern derivative, cocaine, has important medical use as a local anesthetic. Unfortunately, its increasing abuse in the 1980s clearly has reached epidemic proportions.

The purpose of this series is to explore in depth the psychological and behavioral effects that psychoactive drugs have on the individual, and also, to investigate the ways in which drug use influences the legal, economic, cultural, and even moral aspects of societies. The information presented here (and in other books in this series) is based on many clinical and laboratory studies and other observations by people from diverse walks of life.

Over the centuries, novelists, poets, and dramatists have provided us with many insights into the sometimes seductive but ultimately problematic aspects of alcohol and drug use. Physicians, lawyers, biologists, psychologists, and social scientists have contributed to a better understanding of the causes and consequences of using these substances. The authors in this series have attempted to gather and condense all the latest information about drug use and abuse. They have also described the sometimes wide gaps in our knowledge and have suggested some new ways to answer many difficult questions.

One such question, for example, is how do alcohol and drug problems get started? And what is the best way to treat them when they do? Not too many years ago, alcoholics and drug abusers were regarded as evil, immoral, or both. It is now recognized that these persons suffer from very complicated diseases involving deep psychological and social problems. To understand how the disease begins and progresses, it is necessary to understand the nature of the substance, the behavior of addicts, and the characteristics of the society or culture in which they live.

Although many of the social environments we live in are very similar, some of the most subtle differences can strongly influence our thinking and behavior. Where we live, go to school and work, whom we discuss things with — all influence our opinions about drug use and misuse. Yet we also share certain commonly accepted beliefs that outweigh any differences in our attitudes. The authors in this series have tried to identify and discuss the central, most crucial issues concerning drug use and misuse.

Despite the increasing sophistication of the chemical substances we create in the laboratory, we have a long way to go in our efforts to make these powerful drugs work for us rather than against us.

The volumes in this series address a wide range of timely questions. What influence has drug use had on the arts? Why do so many of today's celebrities and star athletes use drugs, and what is being done to solve this problem? What is the relationship between drugs and crime? What is the physiological basis for the power drugs can hold over us? These are but a few of the issues explored in this far-ranging series.

Educating people about the dangers of drugs can go a long way towards minimizing the desperate consequences of substance abuse for individuals and society as a whole. Luckily, human beings have the resources to solve even the most serious problems that beset them, once they make the commitment to do so. As one keen and sensitive observer, Dr. Lewis Thomas, has said,

> There is nothing at all absurd about the human condition. We matter. It seems to me a good guess, hazarded by a good many people who have thought about it, that we may be engaged in the formation of something like a mind for the life of this planet. If this is so, we are still at the most primitive stage, still fumbling with language and thinking, but infinitely capacitated for the future. Looked at this way, it is remarkable that we've come as far as we have in so short a period, really no time at all as geologists measure time. We are the newest, youngest, and the brightest thing around.

NUTRITION & THE BRAIN

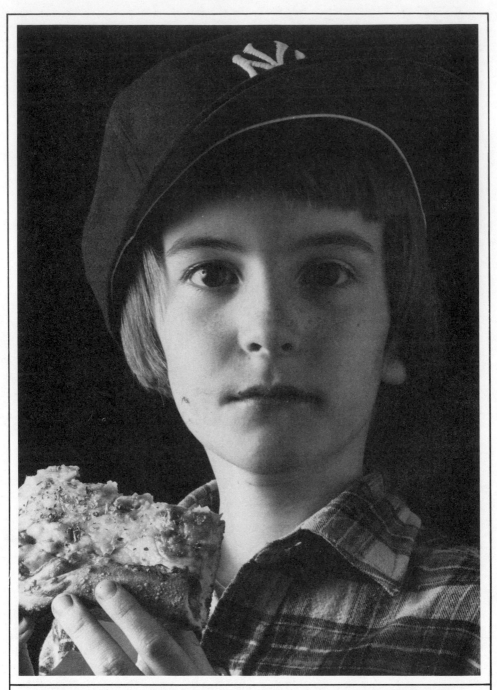

Sometimes the chemical activity in the brain may trigger a desire for particular foods. A person who wants to relax, for example, may crave carbohydrate-rich foods, such as pizza.

CHAPTER 1

DIET AND THE BRAIN

Do you remember the old saw, "You are what you eat"? Well, it's truer than you thought. There is a revolutionary idea in brain science. What you eat can affect how you think and how you act: whether you are alert or sleepy, whether you are sad or elated, whether you can study efficiently or not.

If a neuroscientist had heard such ideas during the 1960s, his or her immediate reaction would have been, "Impossible." No one believed that the activity of the brain could be influenced by the food we eat. But that is all changing. Scientists are doing experiments to see whether they can treat mental conditions with food components. Research suggests that it might do some good to eat foods rich in carbohydrates when you want to relax or have a high-protein snack when it is important to be alert. There is solid evidence that changes in the diet can produce changes in brain chemistry and function in a matter of minutes.

The Blood-Brain Barrier

There were excellent reasons for the skepticism of science earlier in this century regarding the effects of food on behavior. The most compelling of these concerned the existence of what is called the blood-brain barrier, a specialized

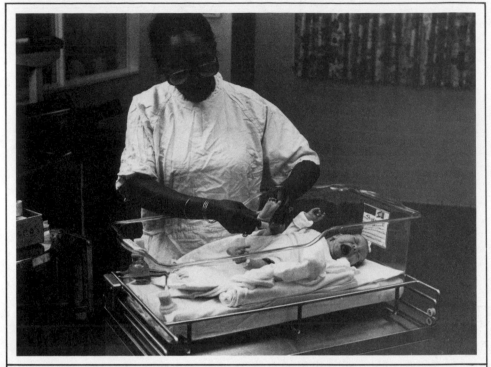

A blood sample taken from this baby will be tested for phenylketonuria (PKU), a serious genetic disease. If the condition is discovered early, a special diet can prevent it from harming the child.

layer of cells that insulates and protects the brain from many substances in the blood, and also from changes in blood chemistry.

The cells that make up the blood-brain barrier protect the brain by excluding all but a select few substances from entering the brain and the spinal cord. Until recently, it was thought that the basic nutrients in food — the amino acids that make up proteins and the carbohydrates in starches — could get through the barrier only in carefully controlled amounts. All the research indicated that when someone gulped down a carbohydrate-rich candy bar or a protein-rich hamburger, the blood-brain barrier acted to keep the brain levels of amino acids and carbohydrates at the same steady level.

Because neuroscientists thought that the passage of amino acids and other food constituents across the blood-brain barrier was strictly controlled, they believed that chemicals from food could make a significant difference in brain activity only in abnormal circumstances. They knew, for example, that poor nutrition during pregnancy and the early years of life could cause permanent damage to the brain. They also knew of a set of pathological conditions caused by genetic defects that interfere with food metabolism. Persons who have the faulty genes that cause those conditions can suffer permanent brain damage because they cannot metabolize food normally.

Probably the best known of these conditions is phenylketonuria (PKU), an inherited disease caused by a defect in a gene that is essential for the body's processing of phe-

In the first part of the 20th century scientists believed that eating such foods as candy bars or hamburgers had little impact on brain chemistry. This theory has since been disproved.

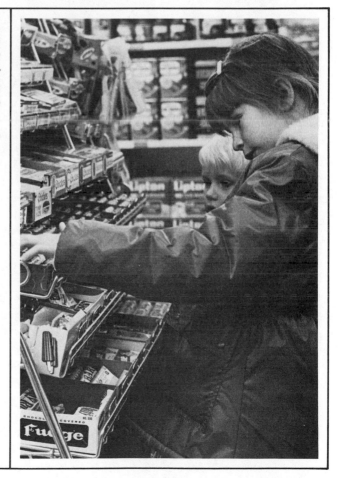

nylalanine, an amino acid found in most proteins. If nothing is done, phenylalanine builds up in the blood and causes severe mental retardation. Every time a youngster with PKU bites into a hamburger or a pizza, he or she sets up a chain of events that causes harm to brain cells. Fortunately, there is now a simple test that can detect this condition in the first days of life. That test is done on almost every baby born in the United States. If PKU is detected, mental retardation can be prevented by putting the child on a special phenylalanine-free diet (which has the one big drawback of being pretty tasteless).

With those exceptions aside, almost no other connection between diet and brain function was taken very seriously by neuroscientists.

The Diet-Brain Connection

The attitude of neuroscientists has changed completely. It is now generally accepted that the chemistry and function of the brain can be influenced even by a single meal. That idea has revolutionary implications for basic research, for medicine, and for everyday life.

In basic science, the newly established link between diet and brain function has opened new areas of research about specific nutrients and diet in general. A number of neuroscientists are studying how amino acids and other food molecules enter the brain and what they do once they get there. In medicine, the diet-brain connection has raised the possibility that simple manipulation of food intake can be used to help treat a number of mental conditions, such as depression, that afflict millions of people. And in everyday life, there is a real possibility that learning how and when to eat the right kinds of food can enable people to sleep better, lose weight, and improve alertness.

Some of these theories are being applied already. Commercially, vendors of health foods are doing a brisk business in what they describe as natural treatments for insomnia and other conditions on which research has indicated that food intake might have an influence. A few books listing what foods should be eaten at specific times of day have been written for the general public. (The basic concept is to eat protein-rich foods when alertness is important, as before an exam or an interview, and carbohydrates when relaxation is the goal.)

Scientists working in the field tend to be cautious concerning the claims being made about commercial products. But at the same time, they are busily exploring a number of possible practical applications of their knowledge. Because human behavior is a complex subject and brain function is even more complex, most scientists are being careful about claims that dramatic changes in serious medical conditions can be achieved by simple dietary alterations. On the other hand, they note that not much harm can come from putting the theory to work in everyday life. If someone eats a tunafish sandwich (rich in protein) to increase alertness or has a plate of spaghetti (lots of carbohydrates) to relax, no damage is done, and some good may come of it.

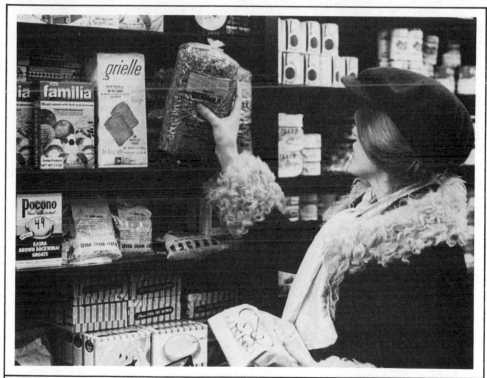

Research concerning the link between diet and mental functioning has inspired health food store owners to promote natural treatments for such conditions as insomnia and depression.

These practical hints about what to eat come from some of the most important brain research in history. In the past few decades, neuroscientists have learned a lot about how the brain functions. It turns out that chemistry, much of it involving molecules found in food, is a pivotal element of brain function.

The Chemistry of Brain Function

Specifically, the link between diet and brain function comes from the understanding of the role that chemicals play in the way signals are transmitted by neurons, which are the nerve cells of the nervous system, including the brain and the spinal cord. A neuron is a long, thin cell that specializes in the transmission of signals. Its major constituents include a long extension called an axon and many shorter branches called dendrites.

Axons and dendrites reach out to link neurons. If you look with the right kind of microscope at a sample of brain tissue, you will see that the brain (and the spinal cord as well) consists of an intricately interlinked set of many millions of neurons, with axons reaching out to dendrites. In the brain, the axon of one neuron may make contact with hundreds or thousands of dendrites from other nerve cells.

Those cells communicate by a combination of electricity and chemistry. A signal is transmitted down an axon in the form of an electrical wave. When a pin pricks a finger, for example, such an electrical wave is stimulated in a pain nerve. Chemistry enters the process when that electrical impulse arrives at the end of the nerve. The signal is passed on to a neighboring nerve by the release of chemicals called neurotransmitters. Every axon has small packages full of neurotransmitters at its end. When the electrical signal arrives at the nerve ending, the neurotransmitter molecules pop out of the axon. They cross what neuroscientists call the synapse, the narrow space between nerve cells, and trigger an electrical wave in the neighboring neuron.

Scientists have identified more than 40 neurotransmitters since the first of the molecules, acetylcholine, was discovered and identified by the German scientist Otto Loewi during the 1920s (see Chapter 3). The study of neurotrans-

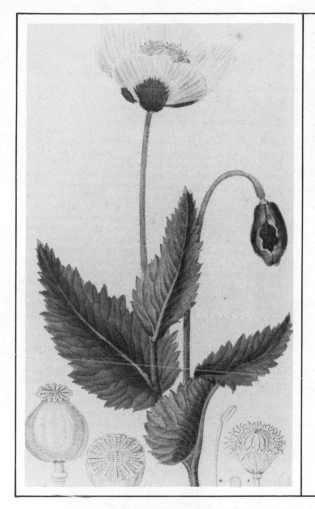

Opium, derived from poppies, was first used for pain relief in the 4th millennium B.C.E. This narcotic acts as it does because its molecules bind to brain receptors for endorphins, which are the body's own pain-relieving neurotransmitters.

mitters, their chemistry and function, how they are made, how they act, and how they are disposed of has become an extremely active field of neurology. This research has in turn produced many discoveries that are important to understanding how the brain works. Many of them have been put to work already.

To give one example, it has been discovered that one family of neurotransmitters in the brain are natural opiates. Called endorphins, these molecules play a major role in the brain's processing of pain signals. They seem to help deaden pain, to cause feelings of elation (the celebrated "runner's high" experienced by marathon runners is believed to be caused by a release of the brain's natural opiates), and to have various other functions.

The discovery of the brain's own opiates has enabled scientists to explain why morphine, heroin, and other plant opiates, which are extracted from the opium poppy, relieve pain and why they can cause addiction. Essentially, plant opiates produce all their effects because the structure of their molecules resembles that of the brain's own opiates. This discovery has given neuroscientists a better understanding of the roles various brain centers play in the way we experience pain. It has also raised the possibility that we can create a more effective and less addicting family of painkillers by producing molecules modeled after natural opiates.

Knowledge about neurotransmitters has been of enormous value in medicine. One example is the treatment of Parkinson's disease, an illness that generally affects older people and that causes progressively worse rigidity of the limbs, tremors, loss of muscular control, and other such symptoms. Scientists have been able to identify the basic problem in Parkinson's disease as a deficiency of a specific neurotransmitter, dopamine, in a specific part of the brain, the substantia nigra. This knowledge led to the development of the drug that is still the most effective treatment for the symptoms of Parkinson's disease — a molecule called L-dopa. This substance can pass through the blood-brain barrier and is used to synthesize dopamine in the brain, making up part of the deficit in the substantia nigra and thus relieving the symptoms of the disease.

Examples of advances in basic research and medical treatment based on neurotransmitter work can be multiplied almost endlessly. So can examples of the misuse of this new knowledge. On the good side, psychiatrists now routinely use drugs to treat schizophrenia, depression, and other mental illnesses. Those drugs are effective because they change the levels of specific neurotransmitters in the brain. On the bad side, unscrupulous chemists working in illegal laboratories have produced dangerous new mind-altering drugs modeled on compounds that are known to affect certain brain neurotransmitters.

A major part of neurotransmitter research concentrates on the mechanism by which these molecules act on neurons. Roughly speaking, that mechanism can be compared to a lock and key. The neurotransmitter is the key. The lock into which it fits is a matching molecule, called a receptor, in the membrane of a neuron. A neurotransmitter will trigger a response in a neuron only if that neuron has receptors for the specific neurotransmitter. Some of the most important advances in the study of neurotransmitters have come from the identification of receptors in nerve cells from various parts of the brain. By studying the location of receptors, neuroscientists have been able to identify specific brain centers involved in such basic functions as hunger, thirst, and sleep, and to gain other valuable information.

For example, we now know that morphine and other plant opiates relieve pain because they have a greater affinity for specific receptors in the brain than do the brain's own natural opiates. By contrast, the powerful hallucinatory effects of the psychedelic drug lysergic acid diethylamide (LSD) are believed to be related to the drug's ability to block brain-cell receptors for the neurotransmitter serotonin, although it is not yet clear exactly why that serotonin-blocking activity produces such bizarre effects on the mind.

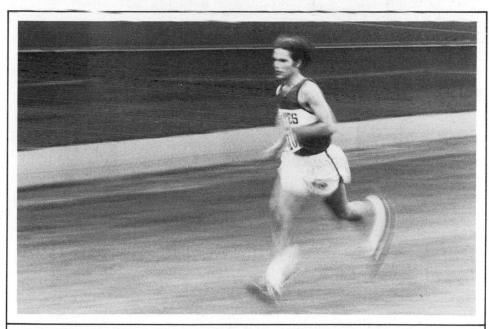

Experienced runners often are able to continue running through pain and achieve a feeling of well-being. Strenuous exercise releases endorphins, causing this "runner's high."

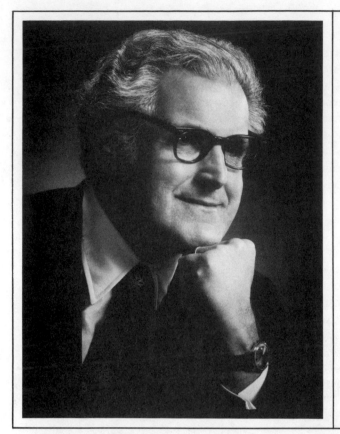

Dr. George Cotzias treated victims of Parkinson's disease with chemical supplements that are transformed into the neurotransmitter dopamine in the brain. Neurons that use dopamine are destroyed in patients who have this disease.

To understand the key, you have to understand the lock. Thus the work on the activity of neurotransmitters (the keys that open nerve-cell activity) and the location of receptors for them (the locks that must be activated to open doors) continues.

Chemical Building Blocks

All this basic research on brain chemistry has a trail that eventually leads to food. The link between diet and brain activity begins with the knowledge that certain foods contain compounds that are, in formal language, precursors of neurotransmitters — that is, they are the starting material that the body uses to manufacture certain neurotransmitters.

One star of this chemistry show is choline, a chemical found in soybeans, liver, eggs, and other foods. You have almost certainly consumed choline today because it is found in lecithin, a chemical used as an emulsifier (a substance that keeps ingredients from separating) in many food products. Choline is a precursor of the neurotransmitter acetylcholine, which, as we shall see, is involved in several interesting brain functions.

Your diet today almost certainly contained tryptophan, another precursor of a brain neurotransmitter. Tryptophan is what the body uses as the starting material for production of serotonin, a neurotransmitter found in many brain centers. Chemically, tryptophan is an amino acid, which means that it is found in most proteins.

Another amino acid that you ate today is tyrosine, also a common constituent of food proteins. Tyrosine is a precursor of the neurotransmitter norepinephrine, which plays many roles in the brain and body.

The idea that we eat chemicals that can be made into neurotransmitters is not especially new. Indeed, the chemical relationships between neurotransmitter molecules and food ingredients such as choline and tryptophan have been known for years. What is new is the idea that consumption of such common ingredients of the diet might affect neurotransmitter levels in the brain.

Breakthroughs in Neurochemical Research

The idea that precursor levels could affect neurotransmitter levels received serious consideration only when research was able to discover a mechanism by which substances from food could pass through the blood-brain barrier. From the point of view of both pure logic and practical experience, the existence of such a mechanism did not seem probable. In fact, changes in brain chemistry caused by changes in the diet seemed to be exactly what the blood-brain barrier existed to prevent. Logically, it seemed unlikely that the brain could function properly if levels of important neurotransmitters such as acetylcholine and serotonin rose and fell rapidly with each meal. It was believed that such rapid fluctuations would cause unacceptable alterations in basic mental functions.

Practically speaking, the example of dopamine and Parkinson's disease appeared to support this view. The discovery that a deficiency of dopamine in the brain was responsible for the symptoms of Parkinson's disease did not lead immediately to an effective treatment, because dopamine does not pass the blood-brain barrier. It was only in the 1970s, when George C. Cotzias, a physician at Brookhaven National Laboratory, found that a related chemical, L-dopa, could pass the blood-brain barrier and that it could be used to form dopamine in the brain, that dopamine-supplementing drug therapy for Parkinsonism became possible.

Acceptance of the relationship between diet and brain neurotransmitters has come about primarily because of the work done in the laboratory of Richard J. Wurtman and his collaborators at the Massachusetts Institute of Technology. In a series of animal experiments that began in the early 1970s, Wurtman and his colleagues (including his wife, biologist Judith Wurtman) provided evidence of a mechanism by which molecules from food can penetrate the blood-brain barrier. The same research has indicated that the presence of varying quantities of a number of different neurotransmitter precursors can influence the amount of each that enters the brain. Experiments have also shown that the rate of production of a neurotransmitter can be influenced by the concentration of its precursor in the brain.

The exact relationship between food intake and brain neurotransmitter levels is still being explored, as is the possible use of diet therapy for various conditions. It does seem clear that brain concentrations of specific neurotransmitters are related to several normal functions, including sleep, body temperature regulation, and appetite. There is also ample evidence that excesses or deficiencies of individual neurotransmitters are related to such abnormal conditions as depression and such chronic illnesses as Parkinson's disease. Researchers in a number of laboratories here and abroad are trying to find out if and how dietary regulation can be used as a treatment for disease, both physical and mental, and to help influence such normal functions as sleep and food intake.

But before we delve further into the relationship between diet and neurotransmitters, there is an even more basic subject to consider: food and the development of the brain. Good nutrition is essential for normal brain development. Children who are malnourished during the critical periods of growth and development are at risk of permanent brain damage. Many children in developing countries are subject to this risk, but it is also present in the United States, where economic and nutritional extremes can be found. Realizing that malnutrition during early childhood can have severe effects on the developing brain, researchers have tried to identify the period of vulnerability to malnutrition, so that more effective measures to prevent brain damage can be taken.

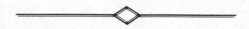

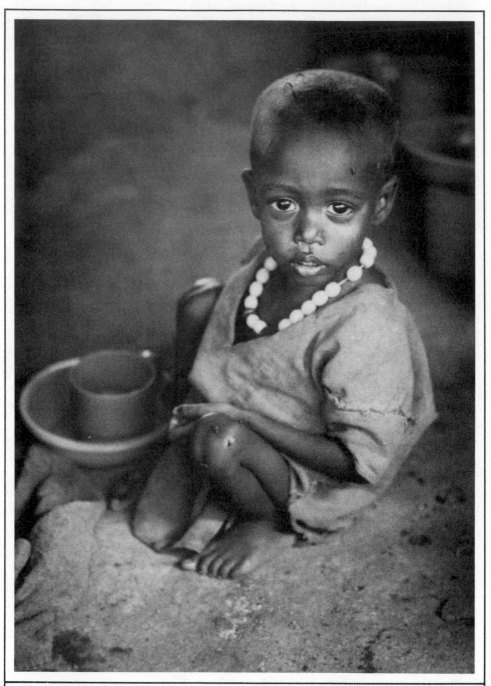

An Ethiopian child awaits a meal provided by a relief program. Although malnutrition can damage a young child's development, proper care later on can do much to compensate for early disadvantages.

CHAPTER 2

MALNUTRITION AND THE BRAIN

Scientists have known for decades that malnutrition is bad for the developing brain. Their studies have shown that when pregnant women eat inadequate diets or when children are malnourished during the first years of life, the result is often some degree of mental retardation or behavioral problems —reading difficulties, for example.

But it has not been easy to describe exactly how malnutrition interferes with the normal process of brain development in humans. One reason is that troubles do not come singly. The child who suffers from malnutrition is also likely to experience other disadvantages. We know that the physical development of the brain is only part of the human story. Human behavior and intelligence are strongly influenced by social factors as well. Parents who cannot afford to buy enough food during pregnancy or to feed their children properly generally live in bad housing, have poor medical care, and do not have many other social or cultural advantages. In addition, their children often do not receive the intellectual stimulation of most middle-class children. It has been a continuing challenge for researchers to distinguish between the physical damage that malnutrition does to the brain and the cultural effects of poverty.

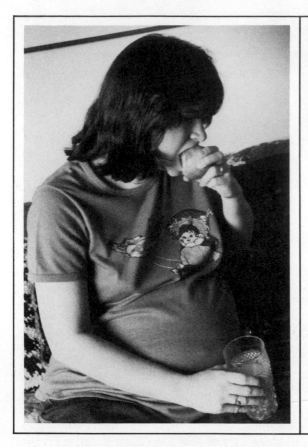

A balanced diet during pregnancy is vital for both mother and child. Undernourished fetuses may be born mentally retarded or develop learning disabilities later.

Another challenge has been to determine the exact sort of damage that malnutrition causes to brain development. Does poor nutrition reduce the number of brain cells, does it interfere with the growth of brain cells, or does it reduce the number of connections between brain cells? Is the entire brain affected in the same way, or does malnutrition damage some areas of the brain more than others? Are there times during development when the brain is more vulnerable to malnutrition? Finally, will good nourishment and enrichment of the environment later in life repair some or all of the bad effects of early malnutrition?

Fighting the Effects of Malnutrition

The answers to these questions are of great practical importance. They determine when a child most needs nutritional assistance and can indicate the most effective remedial measures for malnourished children. Fortunately, a series of experiments on both animals and humans over the past decades has provided many of these answers.

The experiments started with the well-established fact that children who suffer a bout of malnutrition early in life grow poorly and that their brains tend to be smaller than those of well-fed children. As late as the 1950s there was a debate as to whether proper rehabilitation could repair that early damage. In the 1950s a series of experiments provided the answer: yes and no.

Some brain damage caused by early malnutrition can be overcome by good feeding and social interactions later in life. Some cannot. The difference lies in the specific period of early life when malnutrition was experienced, and that difference is due to nature's schedule for brain development.

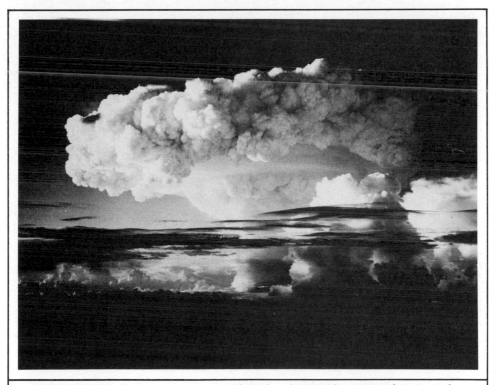

Radiation from American atomic bombs dropped on Hiroshima and Nagasaki during World War II caused grave neurological damage to many unborn children in their first few months of growth.

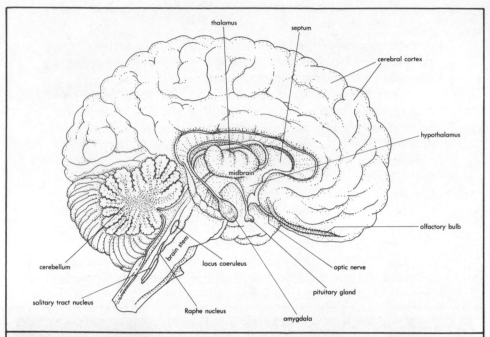

Different parts of the brain develop at different rates. Studies show that malnutrition in the first days after birth is most damaging to the cerebellum, where normal growth occurs most rapidly at that stage.

Neurons, Glial Cells, and the Myelin Sheath

There are two different kinds of brain cells. One kind, the neurons, have already been described. They are the nerve cells that do the actual processing of information and perform the other functions associated with the brain. The neurons in the brain are surrounded by a different kind of cell that greatly outnumbers them: glial cells.

In many respects, glial cells are something of a mystery. They are believed to perform support services for neurons and to aid in interactions between neurons. One function is known for certain. Glial cells are responsible for the formation of an insulating sheath around axons that is made of a substance called myelin. The myelin sheath is essential for proper functioning of neurons. If it is damaged, as happens in the degenerative disease called multiple sclerosis, the results can be crippling.

Work done by various researchers, including John Dobbing and Jean Sands at the University of Manchester in England, has shown that neurons and glial cells have their own separate timetables for development. One very important finding is that brain development goes on well after birth.

It is true that some major steps in brain development take place in the uterus. Studies by Dobbing and Sands in the early 1970s established that the brain develops essentially all the neurons it will ever have during the first four months of pregnancy. Neurons multiply rapidly in a process that begins during the 10th week of pregnancy and ends in the 18th week. These findings explained a phenomenon that occurred after the United States dropped atomic bombs on the Japanese cities of Hiroshima and Nagasaki in 1945. Unborn babies who were exposed to radiation from the bombs between the 10th and 18th weeks of pregnancy were born with defects of the central nervous system, because, as the discoveries by Dobbing and Sands later revealed, the radiation interfered with the normal growth of the neurons.

It is primarily between the 10th and 18th weeks of pregnancy that malnourishment reduces the number of neurons in the brain. But malnutrition later in pregnancy and into the early years of life can affect the total size of the brain by interfering with the proliferation and development of glial cells. Malnutrition after birth can also affect brain function by interfering with the formation of the myelin sheath.

The overall process of brain development does not end with birth. Dobbing and Sands found that glial cells have a growth spurt that begins at the 20th week of pregnancy and continues until about the second year of life. They also found that the myelin sheath forms around axons even later, up to four years after birth. This information has enabled us to define precisely the kind of brain damage that can be caused by malnutrition during pregnancy and early life.

The Timetable of Brain Development

There are some other factors to be considered with respect to brain development. The brain consists of several different centers, each with its individual timetable for development. Neurons in various parts of the brain have growth spurts at different times.

For example, animal experiments have found that the cerebellum, the part of the brain whose functions include coordination of limb movements, begins to grow later than the rest of the brain and that the cells that make up the cerebellum divide most rapidly during the last part of pregnancy. The period of most rapid growth of the cerebral cortex, which is responsible for higher functions such as abstract thought, comes even later.

Therefore, malnutrition that occurs during the critical time for development of the cerebellum will cause problems with the functions it controls, such as coordination of the limbs. If the fetus suffers from malnourishment a little later, the damage is done to the higher thought processes of the cerebrum. One baby might be clumsy, the other a little slow in thinking.

A series of ingenious experiments has helped determine the exact physical mechanisms by which malnutrition causes this kind of damage. One question that had to be answered was exactly how the brain is growing at specific times. It makes a difference if the growth occurs because the number of cells is increasing, because the cells that are already present are getting larger, or both.

Investigators at McGill University in Montreal settled that issue by looking at DNA, the genetic material of human cells. Every cell has the same amount of DNA. That means scientists can know the total number of cells in a brain by determining the amount of DNA in the brain. If the amount of DNA increases while the brain is growing, the number of cells is increasing. If the brain grows but the amount of DNA remains the same, the original cells are getting larger.

Such DNA-measuring studies have shown that every organ of the body, including the brain, goes through three phases of growth. In the first phase, the total number of cells increases. In the second phase, the number of cells increases (but at a slower rate) while cells get larger. In the third phase, the number of cells stays constant while cell size increases.

We know that malnutrition interferes with the normal process of growth because cells are starved of the nutrients they need to multiply and grow. Therefore, the kind of damage done by malnutrition depends on the phase of growth during which it occurs. Early malnutrition limits the number of cells that form and later malnutrition stunts the growth of cells.

We already noted that different parts of the brain enter the three growth phases at different times during pregnancy and early life. In experiments with rats, it was found that the cerebellum, the brain center that controls limb coordination, has the most rapid growth in the number of brain cells in the two weeks following birth. The cerebrum, which controls higher thought, has a slower but longer growth spurt, which ends three weeks after birth. The brain stem, which governs the most basic and primitive functions of the body, has a very slow increase in cell numbers for two weeks after birth. And the hippocampus, a brain center involved in the control of emotions, has its growth spurt during the first few days of the third week of life. Interference with development of the hippocampus could lead to emotional problems later in life.

When animals were deliberately malnourished in their first days of life, the earliest and most severe effects were on

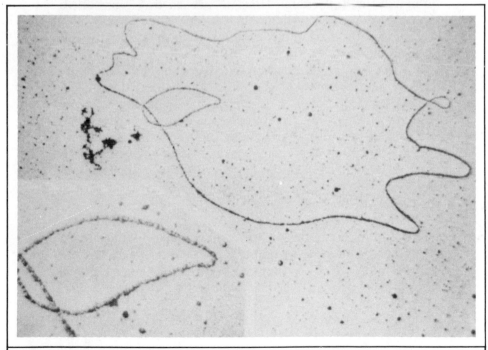

By studying deoxyribonucleic acid (DNA), the carrier of human genetic information, scientists have been able to determine the ways in which malnutrition damages bodily functions.

the cerebellum, where cell division was slowed in just a few days. The number of cells in the cerebrum was affected only after two weeks of malnutrition. Growth in the hippocampus was reduced after three weeks of malnourishment.

But whatever region was studied, one finding remained constant: the more rapid the rate of cell growth, the earlier and more severe the effects of malnutrition.

The kind of experiments done with animals obviously is not possible with humans. But neuroscientists have examined the brains of stillborn fetuses and infants who died of accidents or of disease. They found that the number of cells in the brain increases steadily during pregnancy, with the increase slowing at birth but continuing until 18 months of age. There is no increase in brain-cell numbers after 18 months.

Dobbing and Sands found two major spurts in human brain-cell multiplication. One occurs around the fourth month of pregnancy, when neurons reproduce rapidly. The second is at the time of birth and is due to the rapid division of glial cells.

Measurements of children who were starved early in life gave living proof of the damage done by malnutrition during the critical period of brain development. One kind of damage is obvious. These children have heads that are smaller than normal because their brains have suffered from growth retardation. Postmortem examination of South American children who died of starvation in the first year of life found abnormally low numbers of neurons and reduced myelin sheath formation.

Other studies in animals and humans have found a different and more subtle kind of brain damage. In addition to reducing the number of brain cells, starvation reduces the number of connections between brain cells. Fewer connections between brain cells are believed to hurt the brain's performance.

One such study was done in the 1970s by Bernard Cragg of Monash University in Australia. When rats were starved during the first weeks of life, Cragg found, the number of axon endings, which make contact with other neurons, was reduced by about 40%. Evidence that the same damage occurs in humans comes from measurements of brain levels of chemicals called gangliosides, which are found around the cell extensions that reach out to other neurons. Brain ganglioside levels are abnormally low in animals and humans that are starving.

The Consequences of Malnutrition

By the mid-1970s it was clear that malnutrition early in life reduces not only the number of brain cells but also the connections between cells. The next issue to be settled was the practical importance of these deficiencies on human performance. That issue aroused some controversy because human intelligence depends not only on physical factors, such as the size of the brain, but on social factors such as education, social class, and the kind of environment in which the child is raised. If brain size were the only factor in intelligence, people with the largest heads would be the best achievers, which is not at all true.

An example of how difficult it is to pinpoint the effect of malnutrition came in a series of studies of South African children who had been malnourished in infancy. Their IQs were significantly lower than the IQs of children who had been well fed in infancy. But critics immediately pointed out that the well-fed children came from higher-income families and had better housing, education, and environmental stimulation. It was obviously necessary to do human studies that took different social backgrounds into account.

A more specific study was done in Jamaica, where children who were malnourished early in life were compared with better-nourished brothers and sisters and children of the same age and social backgrounds from other families. The children who had been malnourished had the lowest IQs. Their well-fed brothers and sisters scored higher, and the well-fed children from other families scored highest. In addition, teachers said that the children who had experienced early malnutrition were the most difficult to teach, while friends said they were the hardest to get along with. The Jamaican study did show that social factors played a role, since brothers and sisters of malnourished children shared some of their problems. But it also showed that malnutrition early in life can lower IQ and cause other problems.

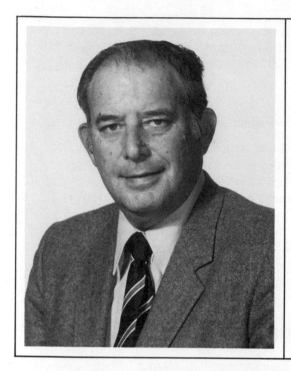

Myron Winick examined the effects of malnutrition on brain development and intelligence and concluded that the earlier malnourished children were placed in a nurturing environment, the better their chances were for eventual recovery.

Perhaps the most convincing evidence of the effects of early malnutrition on brain development was found in studies of Korean orphans by Myron Winick, a physician at the Columbia University Institute of Human Nutrition. The first study looked at three groups of children — one that had been severely malnourished in the first six months of life, one in which malnutrition was less severe, and a third that had been well fed early in life. All the children had been adopted before the age of three by middle-class American families, a fact that minimized the impact of social factors. When the children were tested between the ages of 8 and 10, the IQs of the severely malnourished children averaged 103. The well-fed children had an average IQ of 112, and the children who experienced moderate malnutrition averaged 108. When school performance was studied, the previously malnourished children were found to be exactly at the average for all American children, while the well-fed children were performing significantly above average.

A second study looked at Korean children between the ages of three and five who were adopted by American families. This group did not do as well as the first three groups; the malnourished children in it had IQs below the American average. A detailed analysis showed a direct relationship between IQ and the age of adoption. The children who were adopted at earlier ages did better than those who were adopted later.

The conclusion that Winick and his colleagues drew from these studies is that early malnutrition does harm intellectual performance. The harm is greatest for children who are both malnourished and raised in poor conditions. But an improved environment can compensate for that damage to some extent, and the earlier a child is moved into a better situation, the better the outcome will be. As Winick summed it up, there is "an interaction between malnutrition and the whole poverty cycle, an interaction that somehow results in permanent developmental retardation."

The damage done by malnutrition on brain development is well established. But this effect of diet on the brain takes place early in life. What about the effects of nutrition on the brain later in life — the effect of daily diet on brain chemistry and function? This is a relatively new field, but after two decades of research, a great deal of information about how the foods we eat affect the way our brains operate has emerged.

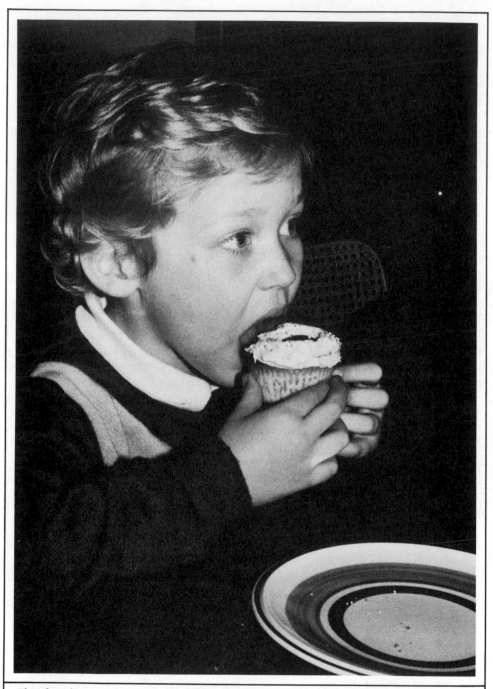

The foods people eat can affect the chemical function of brain cells. A cupcake, rich in carbohydrates, will stimulate the body to release insulin, which in turn causes cells to absorb sugar and amino acids.

CHAPTER 3

NUTRITION AND BRAIN CHEMISTRY

To understand how the food we eat can affect brain function, we must first understand the chemistry of neurotransmitters, the compounds that transmit signals from one neuron to another.

As mentioned in Chapter 1, some 40 different compounds have been identified as neurotransmitters, and the number is still growing. Chemically, neurotransmitters are a diverse group. The neurotransmitters that will interest us most in this book include some relatively simple molecules called amino acids. Every time you eat protein, you ingest amino acids, because a protein is a long molecule that consists of many connected amino acids.

Other neurotransmitters are peptides, molecules that are also made up of a chain of amino acids. (The distinction between a peptide and a protein is not precise, but a peptide usually is defined as a single chain containing no more than 10 amino acids, whereas a protein can be a chain of more than 10 amino acids or several linked chains.) Still other neurotransmitters are classified as catecholamines, a name indicating that each of them contains the chemical group called an amine. Other chemicals in the general amine family are also neurotransmitters; histamine is one of them and serotonin is another. These are described in greater detail later.

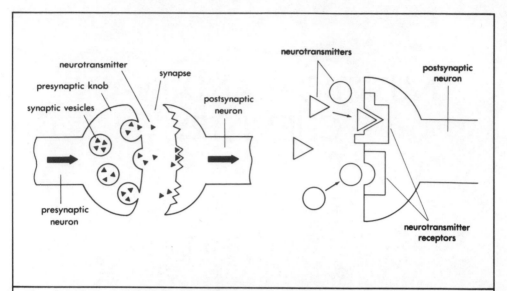

The drawing on the left shows how one neuron signals another across the synapse between them by emitting neurotransmitters. The illustration on the right shows how each kind of neurotransmitter fits only one kind of receptor on the target neuron.

Despite the fact that they are chemically diverse, neurotransmitters have a number of things in common — specifically, the way they are reduced and disposed of in the body. All neurotransmitters are produced from starting materials (precursors, to use the formal term) that are commonly available in the body. They are manufactured (synthesized is the term biologists prefer) in a series of steps by enzymes, which are proteins that promote chemical reactions in the body. For example, peptide neurotransmitters are synthesized by enzymes that link amino acids, the precursor molecules. Of special importance to us is that some amino acid neurotransmitters either come directly from food or are synthesized from precursor molecules that come from food.

Most neurotransmitters are made in the nerve endings from which they are released, but some are made in the main body of the cell and are transported to the nerve ending. When they are released by a neuron, neurotransmitter molecules cross the synapse and bind to receptors on the neighboring neuron. Once a neurotransmitter has done its job, it

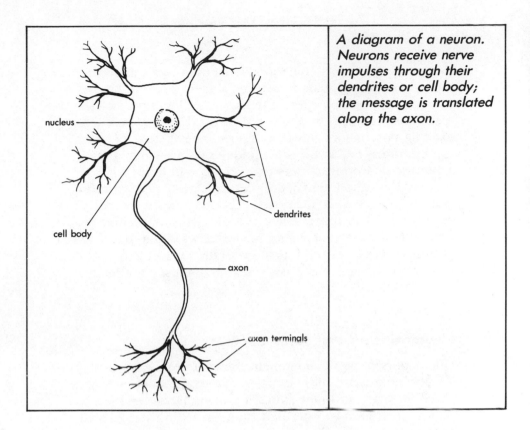

A diagram of a neuron. Neurons receive nerve impulses through their dendrites or cell body; the message is translated along the axon.

nucleus

cell body

dendrites

axon

axon terminals

has to be removed. The body has several ways to dispose of neurotransmitters. In some cases, they are destroyed by enzymes in the synapse, the space between nerve cells. In other cases, they are absorbed by glial cells. Most of the time, however, neurotransmitters are pumped back into the neuron that released them so that they can be used again.

The simple picture described in the last few paragraphs is based on knowledge that took several decades of intensive research to uncover. This laboratory work has been responsible for some of the most striking advances in drug therapy. For example, it is known that one widely used group of antidepressant drugs relieves depression by inhibiting the activity of monoamine oxidase, the enzyme that degrades neurotransmitters used by neurons in brain centers concerned with emotion. By interfering with the destruction of the neurotransmitter, the drugs increase the neurotransmitters' activity and therefore change brain function. Another family of antidepressants increases the activity of these neurotransmitters in a different way — by preventing their inactivation. Reserpine, a compound used both as a tranquilizer and to reduce high blood pressure, acts by causing the neurotransmitter norepinephrine to leak out of neurons into the space between cells, where it is destroyed by enzymes. One exciting point about this research on mental state and neurotransmitters is that the same findings are now being made about the neurotransmitters that originate in food.

But this description of drug research makes it seem more efficient than it was. It implies that the drugs were put to use because researchers knew of their effect on neurotransmitters. In fact, what happened in most cases is that the effects of drugs were discovered first, generally by accident, and it was only years later that basic research disclosed the reasons for their effects.

Neurotransmitters' Complex Roles

One important point about neurotransmitter research is that a single neurotransmitter rarely if ever has a single activity. If we look at the brain alone, a neurotransmitter such as dopamine is found to be used by neurons in various brain centers controlling different functions. In addition, most compounds that act as neurotransmitters also have very different effects. To give one simple example, histamine serves as a neurotransmitter in brain centers that regulate emotional behavior. It also governs the release of acid by cells that line the stomach and acts on other cells in the nose and elsewhere to cause the uncomfortable symptoms of the common cold and allergies.

If you ever have an ulcer, you probably will take an antihistamine that is designed to reduce the secretion of stomach acid. When you have a cold or hay fever, you take a different kind of antihistamine, one that acts on the cells that cause the aggravating symptoms of those conditions. The practical importance of these multiple functions is that researchers are challenged to separate the varied effects of a single neurotransmitter — to maximize the desirable ones and minimize the undesirable ones. One curious example is that the antihistamines used for allergies also act on the brain, causing drowsiness, while the antihistamines used to treat ulcers do not.

Acetylcholine

We can form a good picture of the complex nature of neurotransmitter activity by examining acetylcholine. That is a logical place to start because acetylcholine was not only the very first neurotransmitter to have been discovered but also is probably the most common neurotransmitter, found in up to 15% of the body's nerve cells. Acetylcholine is also one of the central nervous system neurotransmitters whose concentration has been found to be affected directly by diet.

The acetylcholine story began in the 1920s when Otto Loewi, a German pharmacologist, began studying the vagus nerve, which runs from the brain stem to the heart and plays a major role in controlling the beating of the heart. By exposing heart tissue to fluid containing secretions of the vagus nerve, Loewi was able to show that a chemical secreted by the nerve slowed the contraction of the heart muscle. It took him several years after this experiment to isolate acetylcholine and to show that it was what we now call a neurotransmitter. Other researchers building on Loewi's achievement later discovered how acetylcholine is synthesized and recycled in the body, a subject of interest to us, as we have noted, because acetylcholine is one of the neurotransmitters whose activity is affected by diet.

Acetylcholine is synthesized in nerve cells in a single step by an enzyme called choline acetyltransferase. Most enzymes have long and complex names because by scientific custom their activity is described as specifically as possible. In this case, the name of the enzyme tells us that it promotes a chemical reaction between choline and acetyl — or, more exactly, acetyl coenzyme A, which is an activated form of acetic acid, the chief acid of vinegar. Acetyl coenzyme A is plentiful in the body; it plays a major role in the sequence of reactions in which food is metabolized to release energy.

After it is synthesized, acetylcholine is stored in small packets called synaptic vesicles in nerve endings. When it is released into the synapse and interacts with a receptor on a neighboring neuron, acetylcholine is quickly broken down into its two constituents by an enzyme called acetylcholinesterase. The choline produced in this way is taken up by the neuron and is thus available for the production of new acetylcholine molecules.

Until the 1960s, the prevailing concept of this cycle of acetylcholine production and breakdown was that it was carefully controlled by a natural mechanism to keep the supply of acetylcholine within narrow limits. The idea was that the body controlled acetylcholine levels the same way that a thermostat controls a furnace. The furnace heats the house. When the temperature rises above a preset level, the thermostat turns off the furnace; when the temperature drops below a preset level, the thermostat turns the furnace on. The control mechanisms in the body are complex, but the principle is the same: When the concentration of a substance rises or falls above given levels, its production starts or stops.

There was no reason to believe that the production of acetylcholine by neurons in the brain would increase when blood levels of choline went up after a meal. Indeed, most studies of body chemicals pointed in exactly the other di-

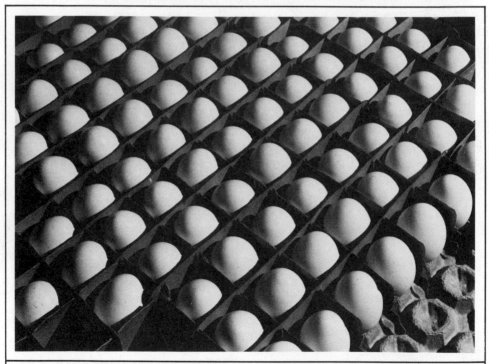

Eggs are a chief source of cholesterol, which is vital to the production of sex hormones. Interestingly, the synthesis of these hormones does not increase when cholesterol levels go up after a meal.

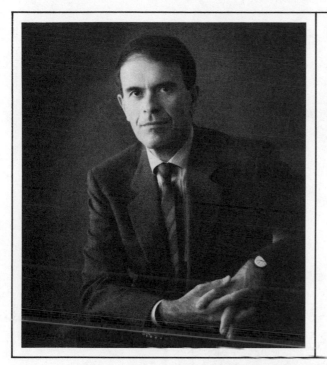

Richard Wurtman and a team of scientists have done extensive research on the link between chemicals found in certain foods and the synthesis of specific neurotransmitters.

rection. For example, many hormones, including the sex hormones testosterone and estrogen, are made from cholesterol, which is found in many foods. Yet the synthesis of these hormones does not increase when blood cholesterol levels go up after a meal. The body's control mechanisms act to keep sex hormone production in line with needs.

To be technical, we could say that production of estrogen, testosterone, and other hormones that use cholesterol as a precursor is controlled by a closed feedback loop. The rate of production does not depend on the amount of precursor material available. Instead, it depends on the concentration of the hormones in the blood. In the same way, the operation of a thermostat-controlled furnace depends on temperature, not the amount of fuel available.

It was, therefore, a great surprise to find that synthesis of acetylcholine and some other neurotransmitters is not controlled by a closed feedback loop. That discovery was made by Richard Wurtman and others at the Massachusetts Institute of Technology in the late 1960s and early 1970s, and its implications are still being explored.

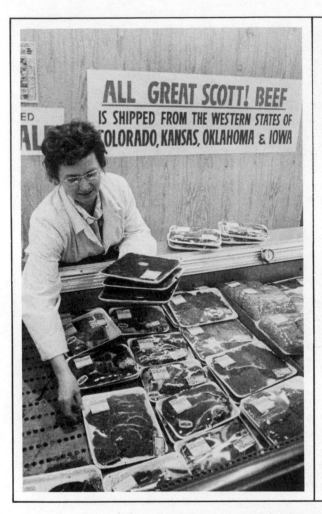

ALL GREAT SCOTT! BEEF
IS SHIPPED FROM THE WESTERN STATES OF
COLORADO, KANSAS, OKLAHOMA & IOWA

Red meat is a major source of protein, which contains some essential amino acids involved in the production of certain neurotransmitters.

The first step in the discovery was the finding that blood levels of amino acids outside the brain commonly rose and fell sharply after meals. Wurtman and his colleagues found that when someone ate a protein-rich meal, the blood levels of some amino acids could increase fivefold. By the same token, eating a protein-poor but carbohydrate-rich meal could cause a sharp drop in blood levels of most amino acids.

Both effects were relatively easy to explain. The amino acid levels were easiest. Proteins are made of amino acids, and blood-level changes in specific amino acids were linked to the exact amino acid composition of the protein that was consumed. A ready explanation was also found for the carbohydrates. Just as proteins are made of amino acids, carbohydrates are made of sugars. The body responds to carbohydrate intake by releasing insulin, whose job is to promote the entry of not only sugars but also amino acids into cells. When insulin production went up after a carbohydrate-rich meal, blood levels of amino acids went down.

The next step was to determine whether these changes in blood levels of amino acids had an effect on brain chemistry. (Carbohydrates were not of major concern because they do not seem to act as neurotransmitters.) In one series of experiments, Wurtman and a colleague, John Fernstrom, worked with tryptophan, a chemical that is the precursor used by the body to make the neurotransmitter serotonin. That particular chemical was studied for several reasons.

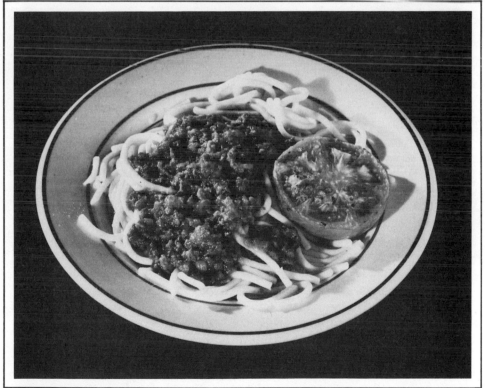

Eating spaghetti and other foods rich in carbohydrates increases the amount of tryptophan that enters the brain, making more of this amino acid available for the synthesis of serotonin.

Tryptophan is found in many proteins, so its blood levels change after almost every meal. And serotonin is of interest because it is involved in depression and other mental illnesses, among its many functions.

The experiments produced an unexpected result. When laboratory animals were given low doses of tryptophan, there was an increase in brain levels of both serotonin and of 5-hydroxyindole acetic acid (5-HIAA), a waste product formed when serotonin is released by neurons. That was expected. But when the researchers fed the animals protein-rich diets, they found that blood levels of tryptophan went up, but the concentration of both tryptophan and serotonin in the brain went down. And when the animals were given meals containing fats and carbohydrates but no protein (and hence no tryptophan), brain levels of tryptophan and serotonin rose.

Carrier Proteins

Something complicated was going on in Wurtman and Fernstrom's work. The explanation came from studies that examined how amino acids are transported across the blood-brain barrier.

As described in Chapter 1, the blood-brain barrier is actually a membrane made up of cells that line the blood vessels of the brain and the spinal cord. These cells transport certain amino acids across the blood-brain barrier by attaching the amino acid to a carrier protein. Once this occurs, the amino acid is carried through the cell into the blood supply of the brain.

It turns out that tryptophan belongs to a family of amino acids that all use the same carrier proteins. They are called large neutral amino acids—large meaning exactly what it says, neutral meaning that they are neither acids nor bases. Tryptophan must compete with the other large neutral amino acids for passage across the blood-brain barrier. Its success in that competition depends not on the amount of tryptophan in the blood but on the amount of the other large neutral amino acids.

A protein-rich meal raises the blood level of tryptophan, but blood levels of the competing amino acids rise even more. Thus, less tryptophan is transported across the blood-brain barrier. A carbohydrate-rich meal stimulates insulin activity, which promotes the removal of most amino acids from the blood. But tryptophan is not as much affected, because it binds to a blood protein that insulates it from insulin. As a result, its competitive position improves. More tryptophan enters the brain, where more of it is available for the synthesis of serotonin.

The Catecholamines and Serotonin

Further experiments in Wurtman's laboratory established the link between diet and other neurotransmitters. When rats were fed choline or lecithin (a complex molecule that normally provides most of the choline in the diet), the production of acetylcholine in brain cells increased. When the rats were fed tyrosine, an amino acid that is the precursor of the family of neurotransmitters called the catecholamines, the production of those neurotransmitters in the brain increased.

However, Wurtman and his colleagues noted some differences in the effects of diet on specific neurotransmitters. An increase in tryptophan levels in the brain always resulted in increased production of serotonin. But adding tyrosine and choline to the brain increased neurotransmitter production only when the neurons that used acetylcholine or the catecholamines were active. The difference appears to lie in the nature of the enzyme systems that produce these various neurotransmitters.

The enzyme called tryptophan hydroxylase, which synthesizes serotonin from tryptophan, is normally available in large amounts. When the supply of tryptophan increases, therefore, so does the production of serotonin. But the enzymes that synthesize the catecholamines and acetylcholine are normally available in just about the amount needed to keep up the supply of those neurotransmitters. Additional supplies of the precursor molecules for these neurotransmitters increase production only when the neurotransmitters are being used up.

Thus far, it appears that only a few neurotransmitters are affected by diet. It seems highly unlikely that the production of the peptides that serve as neurotransmitters is altered by changes in amino acid concentrations in the brain for a variety of reasons, and experiments have not found such changes.

AMINO ACIDS	
Essential	Nonessential
Cysteine	Alanine
Histidine	Aspartic acid
Isoleucine	Arginine
Leucine	Cysteine
Lysine	Glutamic acid
Methionine	Glycine
Phenylalanine	Hydroxylysine
Threonine	Hydroxyproline
Tryptophan	Proline
Valine	Serine
	Tyrosine

Nonessential Amino Acids

What is true of peptides seems to be true of another large family of neurotransmitters, the nonessential amino acids. ("Nonessential" means that the body can manufacture them. There are 10 essential amino acids, which the body cannot manufacture and must get from the diet.)

The nonessential amino acids include glutamate, aspartate, and GABA (gamma-aminobutyric acid). They are probably the most abundant neurotransmitters in the brain. Studies have shown that they are easily produced in large quantities in many parts of the body, so it is reasonable to assume that the same thing happens in the brain. However, not much is known about the synthesis of essential amino acid neurotransmitters in neurons, and it may turn out that their concentration is affected by diet.

So far, the evidence points mostly in the other direction. For example, the precursor of GABA is glutamate, which is in abundant supply in the body. Experiments have shown that even a massive dose of glutamate does not raise brain concentrations; the excess is simply excreted from the brain. As for other neurotransmitters, there are hints that the synthesis of two of them, histamine and glycine, is affected by the supply of their precursors, histidine and threonine respectively, but they are only hints.

Even if only a few neurotransmitters are affected by the food we eat, that effect is still important. The neurotransmitters we have discussed — acetylcholine, the catecholamines, and serotonin — are involved not only in some of the brain's most basic functions but also in a variety of illnesses. Since Wurtman's initial discoveries, he and other researchers have been trying to work out the implications of the relationship between nutrition and brain function.

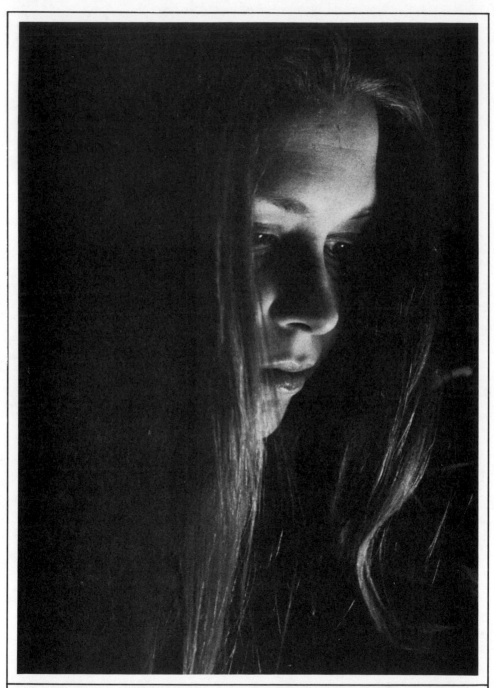

Most people have experienced temporary depression, usually triggered by some deeply upsetting event in their lives. This is different from clinical depression, which is physiological as well as emotional.

CHAPTER 4

NUTRITION AND DEPRESSION

Psychiatrists have known for a long time that sleep and depression are related. One of the prominent symptoms of depression is insomnia. The suffering of people in the throes of deep depression is often compounded by the simple fact that they cannot get a good night's sleep. The new idea of recent years is that there is a biochemical explanation for the link between sleep problems and depression — that both are related to serotonin. It is an even newer idea that both sleep and depression can be affected by the amount of tryptophan in the diet. As we shall see, there is also a theory that several other mental functions in which serotonin plays a role may also be affected by diet.

Let us start with some neuroscience. In formal terms, a nerve cell that uses serotonin is called a serotonergic neuron. All the serotonergic neurons of the brain originate in what is called the raphe nuclei, which are in the brain stem, the most primitive part of the brain. (The brain stem controls such automatic functions as breathing.) These serotonergic neurons send out axons that make connections all over the brain, but particularly in the limbic system.

The limbic system connection helps explain why serotonin-using nerves are involved in depression. The limbic system controls emotion, and depression is an emotion. But serotonergic neurons have many other functions. There is evidence that a serotonin disorder may be present in mental patients who have difficulty regulating aggression. And recent studies have found that some serotonergic brain centers play a role in regulating appetite, obesity, and sleep disorders such as insomnia.

This list of serotonin-related activities demonstrates why researchers have been actively exploring the possibility that tryptophan, the precursor of serotonin (see Chapter 1), might be used to treat a wide range of behavioral problems. The idea is immediately attractive because tryptophan, an innocuous food component, appears to be as safe as any substance can be. The obvious challenge is to prove that something we ingest every day actually has some therapeutic benefit. That challenge is being met. Several researchers have already tested tryptophan in both animals and humans. Those studies have given a reasonably good picture of the usefulness of tryptophan as a therapeutic agent.

Tryptophan and Sleep

Many experiments have centered on tryptophan and sleep. If you drop into a neighborhood health food store, you can see that those experiments have produced positive results, because tryptophan is being promoted actively as a natural alternative to sleeping pills.

As far back as 1967, researchers observed that large doses of tryptophan could affect sleep in humans. Various laboratories since then have shown that large amounts of tryptophan can help bring sleep to normal individuals suffering from mild insomnia ("normal" means their sleeplessness is not caused by serious depression or another illness).

The amount of tryptophan needed to treat insomnia is large if we regard it as a drug but small if we regard it as a food ingredient. Studies generally show that tryptophan in quantities of less than one gram has no effect on sleep, but four grams or more will definitely produce an effect. To show how small that is in terms of food, there are 28 grams in an

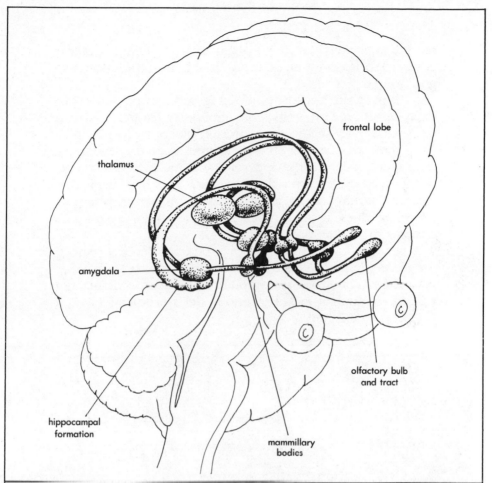

The limbic system is the area of the brain that controls emotion. Scientists believe that a malfunction in the serotonergic neurons that send messages to the limbic system can cause depression.

ounce. To show how large it is in terms of drugs, the standard unit for medications is the milligram — one thousandth of a gram.

If we were talking of tryptophan as a drug, we would say that a dose of 4,000 milligrams helps insomniacs in several ways. For example, tryptophan reduces sleep latency, or the amount of time needed to fall asleep. Another effect is that it increases the total time spent sleeping. Insomniacs who take tryptophan spend less time tossing in bed and more time asleep. One drawback is that tryptophan does not start to work immediately. Its effects begin about 45 minutes after it is taken, so it is best taken some time before the insomniac goes to bed.

Tryptophan has many advantages to offset that slight delay in action. One of its most impressive features is that it does not change the normal pattern of sleep, as sleeping pills do. Almost all drugs that induce sleep reduce the amount of time spent in deep sleep, apparently the most refreshing part of the sleep cycle; tryptophan does not. Another plus is that since serotonin has no negative effect on performance, its precursor does not dull reflexes and slow people down, as sleeping pills often do.

But tryptophan should not yet be considered a remedy for all sleeping problems. Although scientists have shown that it can help in mild and uncomplicated cases of insomnia, the role of tryptophan in more serious sleep problems has not yet been established.

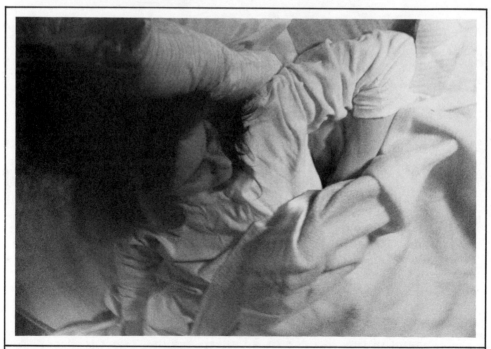

Insomnia has many possible causes, ranging from anxiety to clinical depression. Many people treat the problem with sleeping pills, but these drugs do not produce refreshing, natural sleep.

"It is clear that tryptophan is most effective in normal subjects with long sleep latencies and in mild insomnia," says Herman M. van Praag of Montefiore Medical Center in New York City. "In more severe sleep disorders, its efficacy is less clear. More detailed studies of the efficacy of tryptophan in insomnia are indicated."

The exact mechanism by which tryptophan affects sleep is not known. There is evidence both for and against the belief that it acts by increasing the synthesis of serotonin in brain centers that control sleep. In favor of the serotonin theory are animal studies that found the anti-insomnia activity of tryptophan is increased when it is given along with carbohydrates, which enhance the brain's uptake of tryptophan. More evidence comes from other animal studies showing that damage to the raphe nuclei decreases sleep time, and that when the animals are given PCPA (parachlorophenylalanine), a compound that inhibits serotonin synthesis, they sleep even less. Arguing against the theory are studies showing that PCPA does not block the sleep-inducing effect of tryptophan and that large doses of leucine, an amino acid that competes with tryptophan for transport across the blood-brain barrier, also have no effect.

At this stage of research neuroscientists can only speculate about these contradictory results. One interesting speculation is that the increased synthesis of serotonin in the brain caused by tryptophan intake is only part of the mechanism by which it induces sleep. Another part could be the decreased synthesis of other neurotransmitters, such as the catecholamines, which is caused by large doses of tryptophan. It has been noted that another chemical the body uses as a serotonin precursor, 5-hydroxytryptophan, has no effect on sleep. Unlike tryptophan, 5-hydroxytryptophan does not reduce the production of catecholamines. Further research may help untangle this complex web of neurotransmitter activity.

Research on tryptophan and sleep teaches a useful lesson. When we study sleep or any other function controlled by the brain, we can expect that more than one neurotransmitter usually plays a role. The practical implication of that rule is that dietary measures aimed at changing the concentration of a single neurotransmitter often will not have results that are easy to interpret. Even when we talk about single amino acids, we have to consider that their presence in the

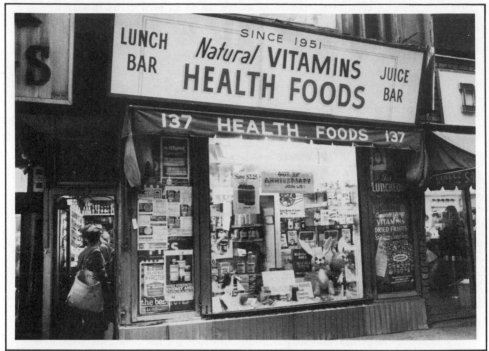

Health food stores sell tryptophan as a treatment for insomnia. Because tryptophan occurs naturally in the body, it is safer than synthetic sleeping preparations, which can be addictive.

brain depends on a sort of competition in which the concentration of one amino acid in the blood can affect the rate at which several others get into the brain.

The Origins and Causes of Depression

Lessons learned from the exploration of tryptophan's effect on sleep can logically be applied in research on the link between tryptophan and depression. This link is not clearly understood, but there are many reasons to believe it exists. One reason is that serotonin is known to be involved in depression. So is norepinephrine, a catecholamine neurotransmitter. We have already seen that doses of tryptophan can influence the synthesis of both serotonin and norepinephrine. And, as mentioned earlier, sleeplessness is one of the symptoms of depression. Finally, there have been several tests on humans in which tryptophan treatment has helped relieve depression.

But the tryptophan-depression connection is not that simple because depression is not a simple condition. To start with, a distinction must be made between, on the one hand, the kind of depression that everyone experiences from time to time because of a loss or a disappointment and, on the other hand, what psychiatrists call a clinical depression. Clinical depression is not a temporary feeling of unhappiness. It is a mental illness, a mood disorder that can be disabling and that seems to have a genetic component.

Depression is actually a group of mental disorders. Several varieties have been identified. Sometimes patients are constantly depressed; sometimes they swing from an abnormally depressed feeling to an equally abnormal state of elation. But all the varieties of depression do seem to be caused by some sort of biochemical abnormality in the brain — something gone wrong with neurotransmitter function.

There is evidence from studies of twins that the abnormality can be inherited. Identical twins inherit essentially the same set of genes from their parents. Depending on the kind of depression that is studied, research shows that when one of a pair of twins develops the condition, there is anywhere from a 40% to 60% chance that the other twin will also develop depression. (The fact that it is not 100% shows that social factors are also involved in depression.)

Enhancing Neurotransmitter Function

What is the inherited trait that predisposes some people to develop depression? It appears to have something to do with the way neurons in specific brain centers produce or use a variety of neurotransmitters, most notably serotonin and norepinephrine. We can make this connection because research shows that the antidepressant drugs that relieve the symptoms of depression act to increase the effectiveness of these two neurotransmitters. Much is still unknown about the biochemical aspect of depression and how antidepressant drugs work, but we know enough to try to treat depression with tryptophan, which affects both serotonin and norepinephrine levels in the brain.

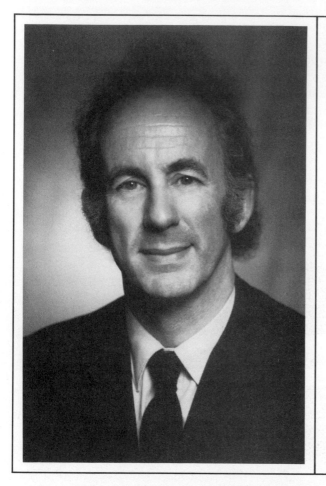

Herman van Praag has used tryptophan to treat both insomnia and depression, with generally favorable results.

Naturally, because neuroscientists are dealing not only with several different kinds of depression but with complex neurotransmitter activities, they do not expect to get simple, clearcut results from efforts to use changes in dietary levels of tryptophan to treat depression. The pleasant surprise is that these studies have found that tryptophan can have a beneficial effect.

Herman van Praag, who was quoted earlier on tryptophan and sleep, has done several of these depression studies, generally with favorable results. In 11 studies that compared tryptophan to tricyclic antidepressants (the most widely used antidepressant drugs, so called because they have three rings in their molecular structures), tryptophan was equally effective in 9 cases and less effective in only 2. And in one large, carefully controlled study in which patients received tryptophan, a tricyclic antidepressant, a combination of the two, or a placebo (an inactive substance), tryptophan and the antidepressant were equally effective (and better than the placebo); the best results were obtained when patients received the combination.

There have been cases in which tryptophan did no better than a placebo. On balance, however, human studies indicate that tryptophan can help at least some patients with clinical depression.

One interesting study done by van Praag combined tryptophan and tyrosine, which is also found in food and which is a precursor of norepinephrine and dopamine, two catecholamine neurotransmitters. The idea behind this study was that because abnormalities of both serotonin and norepinephrine have been found in depressed patients, treatment with the precursors of both might be better than treatment with just one. It seemed to work. When 10 patients who had suffered from major depression for many years were given either tryptophan alone or tryptophan and tyrosine for four weeks, the 5 who got combined treatment improved much more than those who received only tryptophan.

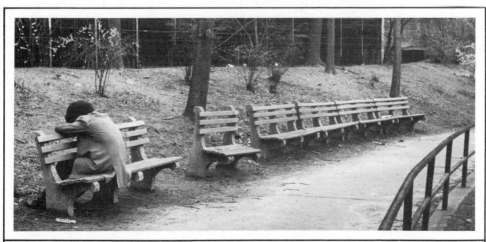

Although scientists have much to learn about the treatment of depression, the use of natural substances to treat this disease can point the way to improved antidepressant drugs.

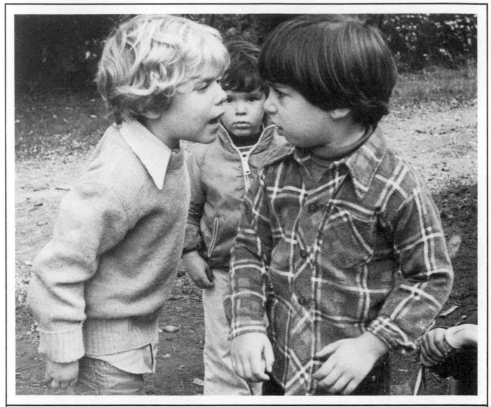

A child exhibits aggressive behavior while at play. There is some scientific evidence that tryptophan may reduce aggression by raising levels of the neurotransmitter serotonin.

Van Praag notes that much of this research on diet and depression is in a very early stage. The same is true of studies in which dietary precursors of neurotransmitters have been used to treat other mental disorders. Tryptophan, for example, has been tried in some patients who exhibit abnormally aggressive behavior. The rationale for the trial is that unusually low levels of 5-HIAA, the waste product of serotonin metabolism, have been measured in patients with aggression disorders. One small study has found some tantalizing indications that tryptophan may reduce aggressive behavior in some schizophrenics.

The most useful results of these studies are the new insights they offer into brain chemistry. For example, scientists working to develop new drugs for depression have generally concentrated on compounds that affect only a single neurotransmitter, such as serotonin. But as van Praag says, since trials of dietary neurotransmitter precursors show that depression appears to be due to an interrelated disorder of several neurotransmitters, "broad-spectrum" antidepressants are more desirable. Although it is still too early to expect that we may someday be able to snap out of a depressed mood by eating the right kind of food, van Praag believes that these studies of diet and brain function could help produce better antidepressant drugs.

There are even more fascinating relationships yet to be explored. At first glance, there might appear to be little connection between depression and obesity. But it has become clear in the past few years that mood and food are closely related, and that changes in diet can influence both. The next chapter explores what scientists have learned about these relationships.

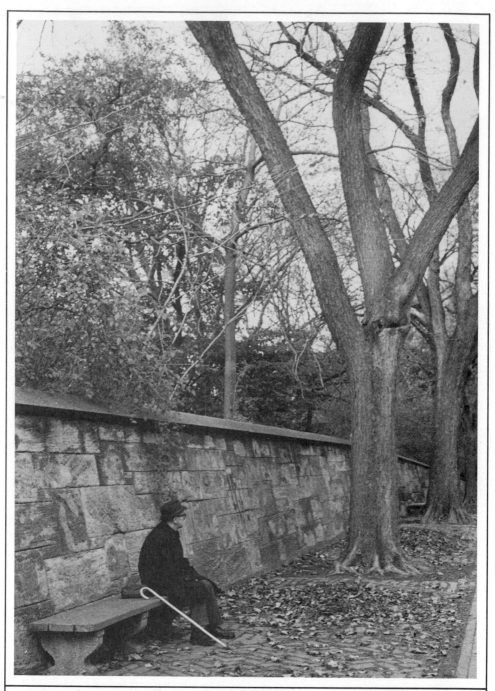

Victims of seasonal affective disorder (SAD), a condition related to low serotonin levels, are subject to serious, sometimes debilitating depression during the autumn and winter months.

CHAPTER 5

MOOD, FOOD, AND OBESITY

Most of us would say that the relationship between food and obesity is simple: If you eat too much, you gain weight. In fact, research over the past two decades has found a much more complex set of relationships between food and body weight.

There is an obvious connection between calories and weight. But there is also a relationship between weight gain and whole classes of foods, such as carbohydrates and proteins. And there is a marvelously intriguing link between specific food components and brain levels of certain neurotransmitters that affect appetite and food intake. Research into these diet-weight connections is a new field, but it has already opened some interesting possibilities about the way people might alter their diet to lose weight and change their mood.

Why mood? Because a large body of evidence indicates that the way we feel affects the way we eat and vice versa. One way to start is by looking at the relationship between food intake and disorders that affect mental functioning in one way or another. In the previous chapter, we noted that people who suffer from depression generally have trouble sleeping. But another major symptom of depression is loss of appetite. And there is evidence that the connecting thread between appetite and depression is an abnormality of the same neurotransmitters discussed earlier — serotonin most obviously, but certainly norepinephrine and others as well.

Fortunately, most of us do not suffer from depression. And many of us would welcome just a touch of one symptom of depression — loss of appetite. We know that serotonin and other neurotransmitters affect appetite in depression, so it is reasonable to think they also affect appetite in persons who are not depressed. We also know that brain levels of serotonin and some other neurotransmitters can be changed by what we eat. Therefore, it might be possible to help control the appetite by eating the right foods at the right time. By looking at abnormal conditions, we can find clues about the functioning of the normal brain.

The Carbohydrates

Scientists have been looking hard at one class of food — the carbohydrates. The simplest carbohydrates are called sugars. If sugars are linked together, they form bigger molecules called complex carbohydrates, which include starch. Dieters regard sugar and starch as enemies in the continuing battle to become or remain thin. There is biochemical evidence to support that view — evidence that some specific neurotransmitter activity drives some people to eat too much carbohydrate under certain circumstances.

Some evidence comes from studies of amitriptyline, an antidepressant drug that often causes weight gain. Amytriptyline is known to affect serotonin brain activity. Some studies have found that patients who gain weight while taking amytriptyline do so because they have an increased craving for carbohydrates.

Those studies are somewhat controversial. But other evidence linking serotonin and carbohydrate craving comes from a specific kind of depression called seasonal affective disorder (appropriately abbreviated SAD). SAD seems to be an exaggerated form of a seasonal rhythm built into the human animal. Poets and songwriters have often noted that spirits soar in the spring. Songs about winter gloom are less common, but we all know the feeling.

Patients with SAD have that gloomy feeling in the fall and winter to a degree that can be disabling. Most of them also tend to oversleep and overeat — specifically, to eat too many carbohydrates. The craving includes not only sugary foods such as candy but also foods that contain more starchy complex carbohydrates, such as pasta and bread. Neuroscientists who have examined the neurotransmitter levels of patients with SAD find that serotonin levels change markedly with the seasons, and that these levels are generally lowest in the winter.

Eating Disorders

A somewhat different and more complex picture emerges when we consider an extremely common eating disorder — bulimia. Patients with this disorder — most of whom are women — go on frequent eating binges in which they eat a tremendous amount, and then purge themselves by taking laxatives and/or by vomiting. Some bulimics also suffer from anorexia nervosa, an eating disorder that causes patients to starve themselves out of an exaggerated fear of gaining too much weight, but other bulimics maintain normal weight while they go through their binge-and-purge cycles.

Both anorexia and bulimia are related to depression; in fact, the great majority of patients with both conditions have a history of depression. In several studies, bulimics have reported that feelings of deep depression often set off binge-and-purge episodes. The overlap between bulimia and depression has led some researchers to treat bulimic patients with antidepressant drugs. Positive results have usually been reported; most patients treated with antidepressants have fewer binge-and-purge episodes.

The bulimia picture is still not entirely clear. We might expect that bulimics would tend to overeat carbohydrates during their binges, because carbohydrate overconsumption can be a result of depression. But researchers have found that bulimics consume protein and fats as well as carbohydrates when they go on food binges. Norman E. Rosenthal, a physician at the National Institute of Mental Health, sums it up:

"We still do not know how the antidepressants exert their therapeutic effect in depression, and it is likely that the mechanism of their antibingeing effect will be similarly elusive."

Researchers study eating disorders because they cast light on normal eating habits. For example, most people show the same kind of seasonal eating behavior that is found in SAD, although in a less extreme form. As far back as the beginning of this century, researchers noted that there is a tendency for people to gain weight in the fall and winter and lose it in the spring and summer. One recent study in Poland found that the best results in a weight-loss program occurred in the spring and the worst results in the winter. And when researchers made systematic observations in the cafeteria at the National Institutes of Health, they found that workers ate more starchy foods, such as cooked vegetables, in the fall and winter, whereas sales of foods rich in fat and protein, such as cottage cheese, yogurt, and milk, went up during the spring months and sales of starches went down.

Diet and Eating Behavior

From the point of view of the average dieter, the way to take advantage of this information is by turning it around. If mood affects carbohydrate consumption, perhaps carbohydrate consumption can be used to affect mood (and through it, total food intake). One interesting aspect of SAD is that the tendency for patients to eat too much carbohydrate is regarded by some neuroscientists as a form of self-treatment for depression. In the 1970s, the scientists Richard Wurtman and Judith Wurtman observed that a carbohydrate-rich, protein-poor meal increased the synthesis and activity of serotonin in the brain. We know that serotonin is involved in depression. Therefore, when a patient with SAD consumes large amounts of carbohydrate, it may be an unconscious effort at self-medication.

Even more interesting to weight-conscious persons was the Wurtmans' discovery that carbohydrate intake is regulated independently of total calorie intake. We mentioned in Chapter 2 that a high-protein meal can actually decrease brain levels of tryptophan (and thus of serotonin, which is made from tryptophan) because it floods the blood with amino

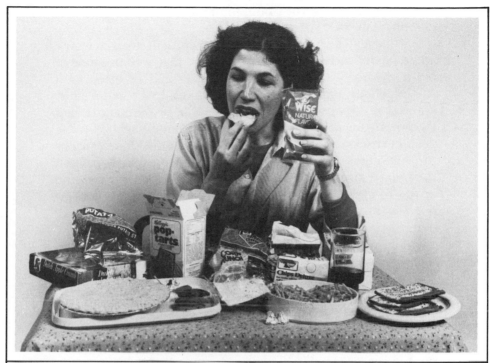

"Binge eating" is compulsive eating for reasons other than the body's need for nourishment. For some overeaters it is part of a binge-and-purge condition called bulimia, which is related to depression.

acids that block tryptophan from entering the brain. Conversely, a carbohydrate-rich meal increases brain levels of tryptophan and serotonin. The Wurtmans, who made this original observation, set about systematically to see if and how the content of the diet affected eating behavior.

They started with a group of volunteers who were overweight but who had normal eating habits. Many of the volunteers confessed that they loved to snack between meals. The Wurtmans set up an experiment in which the kind of food that the volunteers ate at meals and in snacks was watched carefully. The monitoring showed that more than 60% of their snacks consisted of carbohydrate-rich foods.

The Wurtmans were working on the theory that brain serotonin levels had something to do with eating behavior, so they gave these snacking volunteers fenfluramine, a drug prescribed to help people lose weight and known to increase serotonin activity in the brain. Immediately, consumption of carbohydrate-rich snacks went down.

The next step was another experiment to determine whether the carbohydrate snackers ate that way because of brain chemistry or simply because that kind of snack food was readily available. The Wurtmans set up a vending machine that dispensed 10 snacks, 5 rich in protein and 5 rich in carbohydrates. The volunteers consistently passed up the protein snacks, by a ratio of five to one. But the kind of snacks the volunteers took from the vending machine changed when they were given fenfluramine. Although they had the same access to carbohydrates as before, the volunteers began eating fewer carbohydrates and more protein, additional evidence that an internal mechanism was at work.

Interestingly, the Wurtmans found that in their volunteers, the craving for carbohydrates was confined to snacks. At mealtime, the volunteers ate balanced diets containing carbohydrates, fats, and protein. The fenfluramine had a relatively small effect on their carbohydrate consumption during regular meals. In addition, the Wurtmans noted that individuals tended to have a set pattern of snacking. Some limited their snacks to a particular period in the afternoon, whereas others were evening snackers.

On the basis of this research, a theory that ties eating behavior to mood changes began to emerge. We know that serotonin is one of the neurotransmitters involved in depression. We know that carbohydrate-rich snacks can increase brain levels of serotonin. Could it be, as in the case of SAD victims, that the carbohydrate-craving snackers were really indulging in a form of mood-elevating self-treatment?

The Wurtmans had the volunteers fill out forms describing their mood before and after meals. Not all the volunteers had snacked entirely on carbohydrates; some had chosen protein snacks as well. When the answers given by the snackers who craved carbohydrates were compared with those who chose snacks containing both protein and carbohydrates, a pattern emerged. The carbohydrate cravers said they felt significantly more vigorous and alert and were less tired and depressed after a carbohydrate meal, compared with the non-carbohydrate cravers.

On the basis of these experiments, the Wurtmans believe that they have identified a pattern of behavior that could explain why some people eat too many sugary snacks and gain too much weight. That kind of snacking makes them feel good, presumably by increasing brain serotonin activity. Other people can stay away from sugar-rich snacks because they do not experience any pleasurable mood changes afterwards. "Although we do not at this time have any explanation for the difference in mood seen between the two types of obese snackers, these results on the effects on mood of carbohydrate ingestion strongly suggest a disturbance in mood regulation in generating the type of eating behavior seen in these individuals," Judith Wurtman said.

Carbohydrates and Nicotine

Other studies indicate that the carbohydrate connection might have something to do with the often disturbing weight gain that most smokers experience when they give up the habit. Neil Grunberg, a psychologist at the Uniformed Services University of the Health Sciences in Washington, D.C., found that animals given injections of nicotine tended to avoid sweet foods, but sought them out when their supply of nicotine was cut off. He found the same eating pattern in human cigarette smokers: They stayed away from sweets when they smoked, but ate more candy and desserts when they stopped smoking. Another psychologist, Deborah Bowen of the Fred Hutchinson Cancer Center in Seattle, found that smokers who had the jitters when they gave up cigarettes became less irritable when they were given a high-carbohydrate diet. Both studies indicate that post-smoking weight gain could be an attempt at self-medication, with sweets having a calming effect on brain chemistry.

How can we put all these research findings to use in everyday life? One answer is with care, because we are dealing with some complicated matters. The complexity of the relationships between mood, food, weight, and neurotransmitters should be kept in mind when we consider the efforts being made to use dietary manipulation as a treatment for medical conditions and to help improve sleep or to avoid putting on weight. We will look at some of the practical applications of research on diet and the brain in the next chapter.

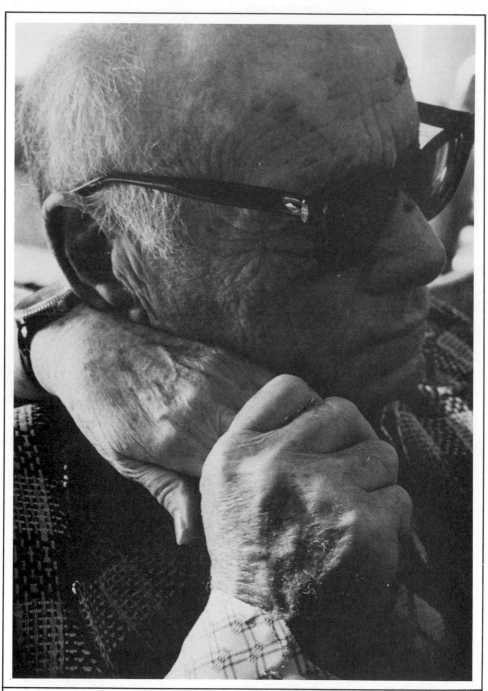

Parkinson's disease, which mainly affects older people, can be treated with certain dietary supplements. Scientists are experimenting with nutritional therapy in connection with some other illnesses as well.

CHAPTER 6

DIET IN HEALTH AND SICKNESS

Are there really "mood foods" — specific things we can eat at different times of the day to induce calm or enhance performance? On the basis of the studies that she and her husband have done, Judith Wurtman thinks there are. She has a set of recommendations for personal dietary management to influence mood and alertness. They are based on three neurotransmitters we have discussed at length in this book.

The first is serotonin, which she describes as a "feel-good" chemical. When we have enough of it we feel soothed and calm, she says; when there is a shortage, we feel grumpy and anxious. The other two are the catecholamines dopamine and norepinephrine, which Judith Wurtman describes as "fight-or-flight" neurotransmitters that increase energy and alertness.

Her formula is simple. Eating carbohydrate-rich foods allows more tryptophan to reach the brain and thus raises brain serotonin levels. Eating protein-rich foods raises brain levels of the amino acid tyrosine and hence increases the activity of the catecholamines. So when we want to be relaxed, she recommends carbohydrate-rich foods such as sugary breakfast cereals (but without milk, which contains protein), bread with jelly or jam, high-sugar and low-fat candies, and pastas with low-fat sauces. For periods when alert-

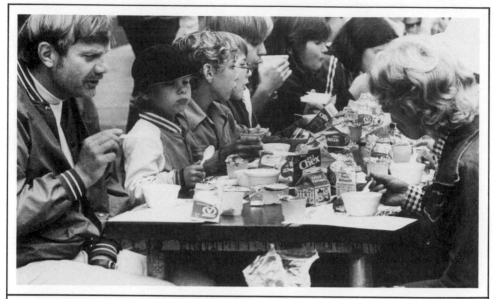

Children and supervisors enjoy an outdoor breakfast. Some scientists suggest that such carbohydrate-rich foods as sugary breakfast cereals induce relaxation, whereas protein-rich foods foster alertness.

ness is needed, she recommends protein-rich foods such as eggs, lean meat, seafood, skim milk, low-fat cheeses, and tofu (bean curd).

A person who wanted to put those guidelines into action would eat a protein-rich meal before a public appearance or any other challenge that called for alertness. Afterward, a carbohydrate-rich meal would help him or her wind down. Carbohydrates would be avoided at lunch, to reduce afternoon sleepiness, but could be eaten at dinner for a calm evening. (Salads and vegetables could be eaten at any time because they do not affect brain neurotransmitter levels.)

These guidelines have not yet been widely endorsed by neuroscientists, on the grounds that the link between mood and food has not been established with enough certainty to make such definite recommendations possible. But there is growing agreement that, in the words of the British neuroscientist Trevor Silverstone, "mood and food are inextricably linked" and that the links are "complex and varied."

The nice part of all the research on diet and brain function is that it allows nonscientists to do their own experiments about the effects of simple changes in eating patterns without doing much harm. Anyone can see for themselves whether a carbohydrate meal helps induce sleep, whether they can fight depression by consuming carbohydrates, whether a high-protein meal will increase alertness.

But it is important to remember that this kind of self-experimentation does not necessarily have any scientific validity, even if everything works exactly as anticipated. Real scientific studies are carefully designed to eliminate any outside influences that might distort the results. Wurtman's recommendations are based on that kind of controlled scientific study. When you drink a glass of milk, thinking that it will improve your alertness, and then find that you feel alert, you have conducted an uncontrolled study that will influence no one but yourself.

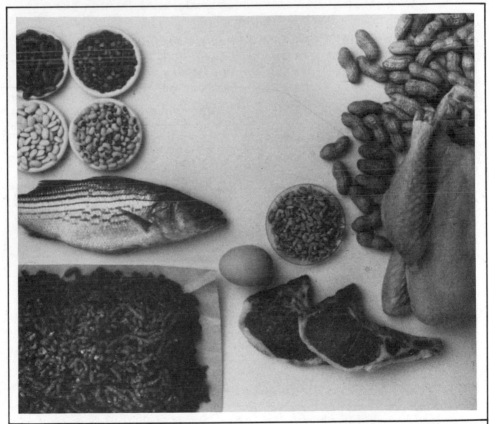

A healthy and balanced diet requires a proper proportion of different foods, including fibers, proteins, carbohydrates, and fats.

Diet and Disease

When neuroscientists do research about the effect of diet on disease, careful controls are vital. One example is the work being done on Alzheimer's disease, a degenerative condition that causes steady deterioration of memory and other mental functions. In the 1970s neuroscientists demonstrated that Alzheimer's disease appears to be related to reduced brain levels of acetylcholine and progressive loss of neurons that use acetylcholine as a neurotransmitter. In the 1980s, when it was discovered that choline in the diet could increase brain concentrations of acetylcholine, it seemed logical to try dietary supplements of acetylcholine precursors as a treatment for Alzheimer's disease.

Several such trials have been made using lecithin (its scientific name is phosphatatidylcholine). The results have been mixed. Some patients who were given daily supplements of lecithin showed improvements in memory and other mental functions, but many did not. At this writing, lecithin supplementation is not established as an effective treatment for Alzheimer's disease.

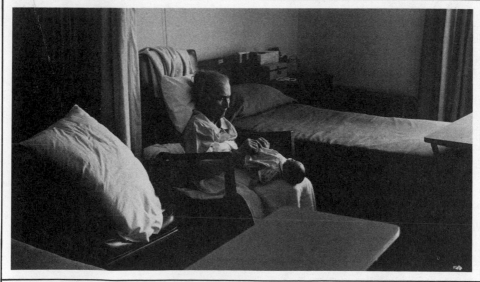

Some scientists believe that Alzheimer's disease is related to reductions of the neurotransmitter acetylcholine in the brain and that dietary supplements can be developed to treat this disorder.

Work is continuing as researchers try to find out why the first tests were not successful. Some hope comes from the history of therapy for another degenerative condition, one that affects physical rather than mental performance — namely, Parkinson's disease, which is caused by a deficiency of the neurotransmitter dopamine. Early attempts to treat Parkinsonism with dopamine precursors failed, and the idea was almost abandoned. It took seven years of work by George Cotzias (see Chapter 1) before he found a way to use the dopamine precursor L-dopa as an effective treatment for Parkinson's disease.

The same sort of inconclusive situation exists in other cases where dietary supplementation has been tried as a treatment for neurological problems. One such disorder is tardive dyskinesia, which can occur in patients who have been treated with antidepressant or antischizophrenic drugs for prolonged periods. Tardive dyskinesia causes uncontrollable movements of the face and tongue. Some studies have found that choline can reduce these unpleasant movements, but most have obtained negative results.

Attention-Deficit Disorder

Tyrosine and tryptophan have also been suggested for attention-deficit disorder, a condition that causes hyperactivity and other behavior problems in children. Stimulant drugs such as amphetamine are the most effective treatment known to control these problems. These stimulants are known to affect brain levels of neurotransmitters, including serotonin and the catecholamines, so it seems logical to determine whether dietary supplements that increase brain levels of these neurotransmitters can help reduce the symptoms of the condition.

One carefully controlled study to test the usefulness of tyrosine and tryptophan was carried out at Ohio State University in 1986. Fourteen children diagnosed as having attention-deficit disorder were given tryptophan, tyrosine, amphetamine, or a placebo (an inactive substance), each for one week at a time. To avoid subjective judgments that might bias the results, the children, their parents, and the doctors who did the study did not know who was receiving what.

Week by week, the parents and teachers of the children were asked to rate their behavior and attention span.

When the study was over, the investigators found that neither teachers nor parents could detect any improvement in the children when they were taking tyrosine. Tryptophan did not show any significant benefit by the teachers' ratings or by the results of standard tests of attention span. But 5 of the 14 pairs of parents reported significantly better results during the tryptophan therapy than when their children took placebo (although tryptophan had considerably less effect on behavior than did amphetamine). The investigators concluded that because tryptophan had virtually no side effects, it might be worth trying when a child with attention-deficit disorder caused more problems at home than at school — during that child's summer vacations or as an evening supplement when the morning stimulant dose wore off.

"Obviously, further study is warranted," they wrote. "This should include manipulation of dosage and long-term safety studies. The latter seems especially important because the trend for 'organic' or 'natural' self-treatment will undoubtedly continue growing in popularity."

Let the Buyer Beware

The self-medication trend is continuing, and not only in attention-deficit disorder. Tryptophan is being sold in health food stores as a natural sleeping pill. Lecithin is being promoted for treatment of Alzheimer's disease, tardive dyskinesia (a muscle disorder), learning disabilities, and Parkinson's disease.

But buyers should beware of this kind of commercially promoted self-medication. For example, few people realize that the lecithin sold in health food stores often contains relatively little of the active component, phosphatidylcholine. One preparation tested by Richard Wurtman contained only 20% phosphatidylcholine and 80% of other compounds. Health-food stores can sell such a mixture because of a federal ruling promulgated in 1938, when lecithin was used only as an emulsifier, to keep the ingredients in such foods as mayonnaise from separating. Lecithin is just one member of the phosphatides, a family of chemicals that share an emulsifying property. The federal ruling allows any mixture of phosphatides to be labeled "lecithin." So anyone who wants to attempt self-medication with lecithin to increase brain concentrations of choline should check for the percentage of phosphatidylcholine in commercial lecithin mixtures.

The big attraction of this whole field is the thought that dietary manipulation has almost no risk and might have some substantial benefits. And as we have seen, some benefits seem to be emerging. But we should remember that the link between diet and brain function is a new area of research and that its findings are always subject to revision. Here is a cautionary tale to illustrate how conclusions can change with time and with new research.

In 1968 Robert Ho Man Kwok, a Boston physician, wrote a letter to the *New England Journal of Medicine* to report a strange set of symptoms whenever he ate in Chinese restaurants: numbness beginning at the back of his neck and radiating downward into his arms, weakness, and heart pal-

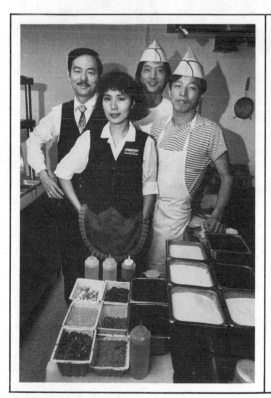

In the 1970s it was thought that the monosodium glutamate used as a flavor enhancer in Chinese food induced a set of symptoms including numbness, weakness, and heart palpitations. It was dubbed Chinese restaurant syndrome. Many experts, however, now believe this syndrome has psychological, not physical, causes.

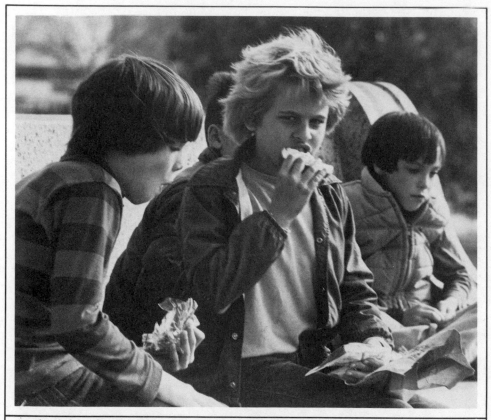

Each child's lunch may affect his or her afternoon attentiveness. Trying to regulate moods through diet probably does no harm, but there is as yet no proof that mood and diet are inextricably linked.

pitations. His report set off an avalanche of letters from other diners reporting the same set of symptoms, which was dubbed Chinese restaurant syndrome. Within a year, researchers said they had identified the cause of the syndrome: monosodium glutamate (MSG), an ingredient used to heighten the taste of food. Chinese restaurant syndrome, it was quickly agreed, almost certainly was caused by the action of the glutamate part of monosodium glutamate on the brain.

Because glutamate is known to be a neurotransmitter, the explanation was accepted universally. Many lovers of Chinese food went out of their way to avoid monosodium glutamate, and many restaurants advertised that they did not use it.

But in 1986 Richard Kenney, a nutritionist at George Washington University, said that his studies indicated that monosodium glutamate did not cause Chinese restaurant syndrome and, indeed, that the syndrome might not even exist. Kenney cited several previous studies, including one in which no symptoms were detected in volunteers who ingested large amounts of glutamate for prolonged periods. But his major evidence was a controlled scientific study of his own in which volunteers who said they suffered from Chinese restaurant syndrome could not distinguish between soft drinks that were laced with monosodium glutamate and those that were not. Some of the volunteers reported that they experienced the symptoms of Chinese restaurant syndrome after drinking some of the soft drinks, but Kenney found that the symptoms had nothing to do with the glutamate content of the drinks. And when Kenney did careful tests, he found that none of the volunteers had any biochemical abnormality that affected the way their bodies metabolized monosodium glutamate. His conclusion: Chinese restaurant syndrome has psychological, not physical, causes.

The last word on Chinese restaurant syndrome and monosodium glutamate has not been said. But the conflicting scientific evidence on the issue illustrates how difficult it can be to draw conclusions about the effects of diet on the brain.

Exploring New Pathways

The challenge now is to find out more about the effect of nutrition on the brain and about the effect of specific dietary measures on mental function. There is a great deal more to be learned.

At the moment, Richard Wurtman says, the only neurotransmitters that appear to be subject to dietary control are members of the monoamine family: Serotonin, dopamine, norepinephrine and its close chemical relative epinephrine, and acetylcholine; histidine and glycine are listed as possibilities. But research has at least set some standards for determining whether diet can affect brain levels of other neurotransmitters. To add other neurotransmitters to the list, they must meet five requirements:

1. Blood plasma levels of the precursor of the neurotransmitter, and of other compounds that affect its availability

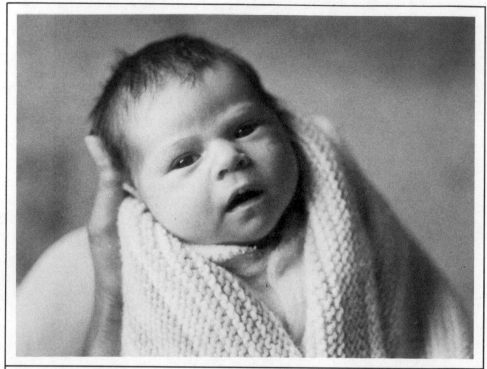

Knowledge about nutrition and the brain is increasing rapidly. By the time this baby grows up, much more may be known about the way foods affect mood, and dietary treatments may cure a new range of illnesses.

to the brain, must be shown to increase after consumption of the precursor.

2. Brain levels of the precursor must be shown to depend on blood plasma levels.

3. A change in plasma composition must be shown to facilitate rapid entry of the precursor to the brain from the blood.

4. The enzyme that controls the conversion of the precursor to the neurotransmitter in neurons must start to synthesize the neurotransmitter as soon as the supply of the precursor increases.

5. The activity of the enzyme cannot be controlled by closed-loop feedback, in which increased concentrations of the neurotransmitter stop its synthesis. Instead, the enzyme must turn out neurotransmitter molecules as long as the precursor is available.

The requirements for identifying neurotransmitters affected by diet sound formidable, but they do set the rules for a whole new field of scientific endeavor. Many more effects of diet on the brain may be added to the existing list. But even if the list gets longer, there is plenty of material for further exploration. Richard Wurtman says: "If, indeed, the monoaminergic neurotransmitters turn out to be the only ones subject to nutritional control, this will still provide the physician and the neuroscientist with a number of interesting mechanisms to explore and explore. . . . These same neurotransmitters are critically important in a large number of physiological mechanisms and pathophysiological states, and are thought to mediate the activity of many neuropharmacologic [mind-affecting] agents. Moreover, they include a number of compounds beside serotonin that could be involved in normal appetite-control mechanisms and in the pathogenicity of obesity."

The study of nutrition and the brain is barely two decades old, but it has already produced a number of major surprises. It is reasonable to assume that the next two decades will see more discoveries and more surprises as neuroscientists explore new paths from food to mental functions. Almost certainly, the best is yet to come.

———————◇———————

APPENDIX

State Agencies
for the Prevention and Treatment
of Drug Abuse

ALABAMA
Department of Mental Health
Division of Mental Illness and
  Substance Abuse Community
  Programs
200 Interstate Park Drive
P.O. Box 3710
Montgomery, AL 36193
(205) 271-9253

ALASKA
Department of Health and Social
  Services
Office of Alcoholism and Drug
  Abuse
Pouch H-05-F
Juneau, AK 99811
(907) 586-6201

ARIZONA
Department of Health Services
Division of Behavioral Health
  Services
Bureau of Community Services
Alcohol Abuse and Alcoholism
  Section
2500 East Van Buren
Phoenix, AZ 85008
(602) 255-1238

Department of Health Services
Division of Behavioral Health
  Services
Bureau of Community Services
Drug Abuse Section
2500 East Van Buren
Phoenix, AZ 85008
(602) 255-1240

ARKANSAS
Department of Human Services
Office of Alcohol and Drug Abuse
  Prevention
1515 West 7th Avenue
Suite 310
Little Rock, AR 72202
(501) 371-2603

CALIFORNIA
Department of Alcohol and Drug
  Abuse
111 Capitol Mall
Sacramento, CA 95814
(916) 445-1940

COLORADO
Department of Health
Alcohol and Drug Abuse Division
4210 East 11th Avenue
Denver, CO 80220
(303) 320-6137

CONNECTICUT
Alcohol and Drug Abuse
  Commission
999 Asylum Avenue
3rd Floor
Hartford, CT 06105
(203) 566-4145

DELAWARE
Division of Mental Health
Bureau of Alcoholism and Drug
  Abuse
1901 North Dupont Highway
Newcastle, DE 19720
(302) 421-6101

DISTRICT OF COLUMBIA
Department of Human Services
Office of Health Planning and
  Development
601 Indiana Avenue, NW
Suite 500
Washington, D.C. 20004
(202) 724-5641

FLORIDA
Department of Health and
  Rehabilitative Services
Alcoholic Rehabilitation Program
1317 Winewood Boulevard
Room 187A
Tallahassee, FL 32301
(904) 488-0396

Department of Health and
  Rehabilitative Services
Drug Abuse Program
1317 Winewood Boulevard
Building 6, Room 155
Tallahassee, FL 32301
(904) 488-0900

GEORGIA
Department of Human Resources
Division of Mental Health and
  Mental Retardation
Alcohol and Drug Section
618 Ponce De Leon Avenue, NE
Atlanta, GA 30365-2101
(404) 894-4785

HAWAII
Department of Health
Mental Health Division
Alcohol and Drug Abuse Branch
1250 Punch Bowl Street
P.O. Box 3378
Honolulu, HI 96801
(808) 548-4280

IDAHO
Department of Health and Welfare
Bureau of Preventive Medicine
Substance Abuse Section
450 West State
Boise, ID 83720
(208) 334-4368

ILLINOIS
Department of Mental Health and
  Developmental Disabilities
Division of Alcoholism
160 North La Salle Street
Room 1500
Chicago, IL 60601
(312) 793-2907

Illinois Dangerous Drugs
  Commission
300 North State Street
Suite 1500
Chicago, IL 60610
(312) 822-9860

INDIANA
Department of Mental Health
Division of Addiction Services
429 North Pennsylvania Street
Indianapolis, IN 46204
(317) 232-7816

IOWA
Department of Substance Abuse
505 5th Avenue
Insurance Exchange Building
Suite 202
Des Moines, IA 50319
(515) 281-3641

KANSAS
Department of Social Rehabilitation
Alcohol and Drug Abuse Services
2700 West 6th Street
Biddle Building
Topeka, KS 66606
(913) 296-3925

KENTUCKY
Cabinet for Human Resources
Department of Health Services
Substance Abuse Branch
275 East Main Street
Frankfort, KY 40601
(502) 564-2880

LOUISIANA
Department of Health and Human
  Resources
Office of Mental Health and
  Substance Abuse
655 North 5th Street
P.O. Box 4049
Baton Rouge, LA 70821
(504) 342-2565

MAINE
Department of Human Services
Office of Alcoholism and Drug
  Abuse Prevention
Bureau of Rehabilitation
32 Winthrop Street
Augusta, ME 04330
(207) 289-2781

MARYLAND
Alcoholism Control Administration
201 West Preston Street
Fourth Floor
Baltimore, MD 21201
(301) 383-2977

State Health Department
Drug Abuse Administration
201 West Preston Street
Baltimore, MD 21201
(301) 383-3312

MASSACHUSETTS
Department of Public Health
Division of Alcoholism
755 Boylston Street
Sixth Floor
Boston, MA 02116
(617) 727-1960

Department of Public Health
Division of Drug Rehabilitation
600 Washington Street
Boston, MA 02114
(617) 727-8617

MICHIGAN
Department of Public Health
Office of Substance Abuse Services
3500 North Logan Street
P.O. Box 30035
Lansing, MI 48909
(517) 373-8603

MINNESOTA
Department of Public Welfare
Chemical Dependency Program
  Division
Centennial Building
658 Cedar Street
4th Floor
Saint Paul, MN 55155
(612) 296-4614

MISSISSIPPI
Department of Mental Health
Division of Alcohol and Drug Abuse
1102 Robert E. Lee Building
Jackson, MS 39201
(601) 359-1297

MISSOURI
Department of Mental Health
Division of Alcoholism and Drug
  Abuse
2002 Missouri Boulevard
P.O. Box 687
Jefferson City, MO 65102
(314) 751-4942

MONTANA
Department of Institutions
Alcohol and Drug Abuse Division
1539 11th Avenue
Helena, MT 59620
(406) 449-2827

NEBRASKA
Department of Public Institutions
Division of Alcoholism and Drug
Abuse
801 West Van Dorn Street
P.O. Box 94728
Lincoln, NB 68509
(402) 471-2851, Ext. 415

NEVADA
Department of Human Resources
Bureau of Alcohol and Drug Abuse
505 East King Street
Carson City, NV 89710
(702) 885-4790

NEW HAMPSHIRE
Department of Health and Welfare
Office of Alcohol and Drug Abuse
    Prevention
Hazen Drive
Health and Welfare Building
Concord, NH 03301
(603) 271-4627

NEW JERSEY
Department of Health
Division of Alcoholism
129 East Hanover Street CN 362
Trenton, NJ 08625
(609) 292-8949

Department of Health
Division of Narcotic and Drug
    Abuse Control
129 East Hanover Street CN 362
Trenton, NJ 08625
(609) 292-8949

NEW MEXICO
Health and Environment Department
Behavioral Services Division
Substance Abuse Bureau
725 Saint Michaels Drive
P.O. Box 968
Santa Fe, NM 87503
(505) 984-0020, Ext. 304

NEW YORK
Division of Alcoholism and Alcohol
    Abuse
194 Washington Avenue
Albany, NY 12210
(518) 474-5417

Division of Substance Abuse
    Services
Executive Park South
Box 8200
Albany, NY 12203
(518) 457-7629

NORTH CAROLINA
Department of Human Resources
Division of Mental Health, Mental
    Retardation and Substance Abuse
    Services
Alcohol and Drug Abuse Services
325 North Salisbury Street
Albemarle Building
Raleigh, NC 27611
(919) 733-4670

NORTH DAKOTA
Department of Human Services
Division of Alcoholism and Drug
    Abuse
State Capitol Building
Bismarck, ND 58505
(701) 224-2767

OHIO
Department of Health
Division of Alcoholism
246 North High Street
P.O. Box 118
Columbus, OH 43216
(614) 466-3543

Department of Mental Health
Bureau of Drug Abuse
65 South Front Street
Columbus, OH 43215
(614) 466-9023

OKLAHOMA
Department of Mental Health
Alcohol and Drug Programs
4545 North Lincoln Boulevard
Suite 100 East Terrace
P.O. Box 53277
Oklahoma City, OK 73152
(405) 521-0044

OREGON
Department of Human Resources
Mental Health Division
Office of Programs for Alcohol and
  Drug Problems
2575 Bittern Street, NE
Salem, OR 97310
(503) 378-2163

PENNSYLVANIA
Department of Health
Office of Drug and Alcohol
  Programs
Commonwealth and Forster Avenues
Health and Welfare Building
P.O. Box 90
Harrisburg, PA 17108
(717) 787-9857

RHODE ISLAND
Department of Mental Health,
  Mental Retardation and Hospitals
Division of Substance Abuse
Substance Abuse Administration
  Building
Cranston, RI 02920
(401) 464-2091

SOUTH CAROLINA
Commission on Alcohol and Drug
  Abuse
3700 Forest Drive
Columbia, SC 29204
(803) 758-2521

SOUTH DAKOTA
Department of Health
Division of Alcohol and Drug Abuse
523 East Capitol, Joe Foss Building
Pierre, SD 57501
(605) 773-4806

TENNESSEE
Department of Mental Health and
  Mental Retardation
Alcohol and Drug Abuse Services
505 Deaderick Street
James K. Polk Building,
  Fourth Floor
Nashville, TN 37219
(615) 741-1921

TEXAS
Commission on Alcoholism
809 Sam Houston State Office
  Building
Austin, TX 78701
(512) 475-2577
Department of Community Affairs
Drug Abuse Prevention Division
2015 South Interstate Highway 35
P.O. Box 13166
Austin, TX 78711
(512) 443-4100

UTAH
Department of Social Services
Division of Alcoholism and Drugs
150 West North Temple
Suite 350
P.O. Box 2500
Salt Lake City, UT 84110
(801) 533-6532

VERMONT
Agency of Human Services
Department of Social and
  Rehabilitation Services
Alcohol and Drug Abuse Division
103 South Main Street
Waterbury, VT 05676
(802) 241-2170

VIRGINIA
Department of Mental Health and
  Mental Retardation
Division of Substance Abuse
109 Governor Street
P.O. Box 1797
Richmond, VA 23214
(804) 786-5313

WASHINGTON
Department of Social and Health
  Service
Bureau of Alcohol and Substance
  Abuse
Office Building—44 W
Olympia, WA 98504
(206) 753-5866

WEST VIRGINIA
Department of Health
Office of Behavioral Health Services
Division on Alcoholism and Drug
  Abuse
1800 Washington Street East
Building 3 Room 451
Charleston, WV 25305
(304) 348-2276

WISCONSIN
Department of Health and Social
  Services
Division of Community Services
Bureau of Community Programs
Alcohol and Other Drug Abuse
  Program Office
1 West Wilson Street
P.O. Box 7851
Madison, WI 53707
(608) 266-2717

WYOMING
Alcohol and Drug Abuse Programs
Hathaway Building
Cheyenne, WY 82002
(307) 777-7115, Ext. 7118

GUAM
Mental Health & Substance Abuse
  Agency
P.O. Box 20999
Guam 96921

PUERTO RICO
Department of Addiction Control
  Services
Alcohol Abuse Programs
P.O. Box B-Y Rio Piedras Station
Rio Piedras, PR 00928
(809) 763-5014

Department of Addiction Control
  Services
Drug Abuse Programs
P.O. Box B-Y Rio Piedras Station
Rio Piedras, PR 00928
(809) 764-8140

VIRGIN ISLANDS
Division of Mental Health,
  Alcoholism & Drug Dependency
  Services
P.O. Box 7329
Saint Thomas, Virgin Islands 00801
(809) 774-7265

AMERICAN SAMOA
LBJ Tropical Medical Center
Department of Mental Health Clinic
Pago Pago, American Samoa 96799

TRUST TERRITORIES
Director of Health Services
Office of the High Commissioner
Saipan, Trust Territories 96950

Further Reading

Lewin, Roger. "The Poverty of Undernourished Brains." *New Scientist*, October 1974.

Nutrition and the Brain: Volume 7. New York: Raven Press, 1986.

Wurtman, Judith. *Managing Your Mind and Mood Through Food*. New York: Rawson Associates, 1987.

Wurtman, Richard. "The Ultimate Head Waiter — How Diet Controls the Brain." *Technology Review*, July 1984.

Glossary

acetylcholine a neurotransmitter that plays an important part in the transmission of nerve impulses, especially at synapses. Nicotine mimics its actions at nicotinic receptors

addiction a condition caused by repeated drug use, characterized by a compulsive urge to continue using the drug, a tendency to increase the dosage, and physiological and/or psychological dependence

Alzheimer's disease a chronic condition characterized by irreversible loss of memory, disorientation, possible problems with speech or balance and decline of intellectual abilities

amino acid any one of a number of organic compounds containing an amino group and a carboxyl; the fundamental building blocks of proteins

amitriptyline an antidepressant drug that affects serotonin activity in the brain

amphetamine any one of a number of substances that act as a stimulant to the central nervous system

anorexia nervosa a psychological illness characterized by a continual absence of appetite

antidepressant any one of a number of substances used to counteract depression

blood-brain barrier a semipermeable membrane that separates circulating blood from tissue fluid surrounding brain cells, thus protecting the brain from some poisons and buildup of unwanted chemicals

brain stem the lower part of the brain connecting the forebrain and midbrain to the spinal cord

carbohydrate an organic compound consisting of carbon, hydrogen and oxygen; sugars and starches are carbohydrates

catecholamines a compound such as dopamine or norepinephrine that affects the nervous and cardiovascular systems, the metabolic rate, and body temperature

cerebellum the part of the brain that regulates muscle movement

cerebrum the part of the brain that coordinates voluntary activity and conscious thought

choline a basic compound found in plant and animal tissues that is essential to the normal metabolism of fats

choline acetyltransferase an enzyme that promotes a reaction between choline and acetyl coenzyme A (an activated form of acetic acid)

corpus striatum part of the basal ganglia, which are responsible for subconscious regulation of voluntary movement

dendrite the branching extension of nerve cells; carries impulses toward the cell body

depression a mental state characterized by despair and extreme sadness; often marked by inactivity

DNA abbreviation for deoxyribonucleic acid, a substance that stores genetic information in certain living organisms

dopamine a catecholamine active in the synthesis of norepinephrine; also acts as a neurotransmitter in the brain

emulsion a mixture in which droplets of one liquid are dispensed in another; often used to disguise the taste of a medicine

enzyme any of a number of proteins that act as catalysts in the body's chemical processes, such as digestion

fenfluramine a drug that reduces appetite; common side effects are drowsiness and diarrhea

glia supporting or connective tissue of the central nervous system

histamine a chemical compound found in nearly all body tissue and released during inflammation and allergic reactions

homeostasis process by which the body's internal systems are maintained at equilibrium

hormone a substance produced by the body and carried by the bloodstream to other organs or tissues, which it stimulates by chemical action

insulin the protein hormone that controls the amount of sugar (glucose) in the bloodstream

malnutrition the state of being insufficiently nourished by proper vitamins and minerals essential to balanced health

metabolism the normal processes in which food is synthesized into nutrient material or used to supply energy in the body

monoamine oxidase an enzyme found in most tissues that triggers the oxidation of a large number of monoamines such as epinephrine, norepinephrine, and serotonin

myelin sheath part of large nerve cells laid down around the axon (nerve fiber); myelin is a complex material that speeds the conduction of nerve impulses

neurology the study of the nervous system

neuron a nerve cell; the fundamental unit of the nervous system; transmits information in the form of electrical impulses from one part of the body to another

neurotransmitter a chemical released by neurons that transmits nerve impulses across a synapse

norepinephrine a neurotransmitter secreted by the adrenal gland and also found in the autonomic nervous system; chemically, norepinephrine is a catecholamine

obesity a nutritional disorder in which excess fat accumulates in the body; generally considered present when a person is 20% over his or her recommended weight

Parkinson's disease a chronic disease marked by tremors and muscle weakness

peptide a molecule containing two or more amino acids

phenylketonuria an inborn defect in protein metabolism that causes an excess of the amino acid phenylalanine in the blood, which can lead to nervous damage and severe mental retardation

phosphatides a phospholipid, or a substance containing phosphorous, fatty acids, and a nitrogenous base, used in a number of bodily processes, particularly the metabolism of fat

physical dependence adaption of the body to the presence of a drug such that its absence produces withdrawal symptoms

placebo a substance that has no pharmacological value but may be effective because of a patient's belief in its powers; often used during drug experiments

protein an organic compound containing nitrogen that is an essential nutrient for humans

psychological dependence a condition in which the drug user craves a drug to maintain a sense of well-being and feels discomfort when deprived of it

receptor a specialized component of a cell that detects changes in the environment and triggers impulses in the sensory nervous system

reserpine a compound used to reduce high blood pressure; sometimes used to treat anxiety

schizophrenia any one of a number of mental disorders usually characterized by hallucinations and delusions, disordered thinking, extreme mood changes, social withdrawal, and other abnormal behavior

serotonin a compound thought to act as a neurotransmitter in affecting sleep functions; widely distributed throughout the body, it acts similarly to the histamines in combating inflammation

synapse the narrow gap between neurons; the point at which a nerve impulse is transmitted from one nerve to another

tolerance a decrease of susceptibility to the effects of a drug due to its continued administration, resulting in the user's need to increase the drug dosage in order to achieve effects experienced previously

tryptophan an amino acid employed by the body in making serotonin

tyrosine an amino acid used by the body in producing catecholamines

vagus nerve a cranial (brain-related) nerve involved in the motor and sensory functions of the chest cavity, heart, and abdomen; involved in swallowing and the sensation of taste

withdrawal the physiological and psychological effects of discontinued use of a drug

PICTURE CREDITS

Courtesy of the Albert Einstein College of Medicine: p. 66; AP/Wide World Photos: p. 64; Art Resource: pp. 10, 21, 23, 44, 52, 75, 78, 80, 82; The Bettmann Archive: pp. 12, 35, 50, 53; Brookhaven National Laboratory: p. 28; Courtesy of Columbia University College of Physicians and Surgeons: p. 42; Courtesy of the Massachusetts Institute of Technology: p. 51; National Institutes of Health Photo: pp. 20, 39; National Library of Medicine: p. 25; The American Red Cross: p. 32; Jean Shapiro: pp. 34, 58, 62, 67, 70, 88; Frank Siteman/Taurus Photos: p. 27; Taurus Photos: pp. 18, 68, 85; USDA Photo: pp. 8, 81, 86
Gary Tong Original Illustrations: pp. 36, 46, 47, 61

Index

treatment of insomnia, 60–62
treatment of schizophrenia, 68
tyrosine and, 67
tryptophan hydroxylase, 55
tyrosine, 29, 55, 67, 79, 83, 84

Uniformed Services University of the
Health Sciences, 77

University of Manchester, 36

vagus, 49
van Praag, Herman M., 63, 66–69

Winick, Myron, 42, 43
Wurtman, Judith, 30, 74–77, 79, 81
Wurtman, Richard J., 30, 51–55, 57,
74–76, 84, 87, 89

Edward Edelson is the Science Editor of the New York Daily News and the past president of the National Association of Science Writers. He is the author of a number of books, including the forthcoming *Woman's Guide to Prescription Narcotics.* He has published extensively in magazines and journals on topics in medicine and science.

Solomon H. Snyder, M.D. is Distinguished Service Professor of Neuroscience, Pharmacology and Psychiatry at The Johns Hopkins University School of Medicine. He has served as president of the Society for Neuroscience and in 1978 received the Albert Lasker Award in Medical Research. He has authored *Uses of Marijuana, Madness and the Brain, The Troubled Mind, Biological Aspects of Mental Disorder,* and edited *Perspective in Neuropharmacology: A Tribute to Julius Axelrod.* Professor Snyder was a research associate with Dr. Axelrod at the National Institutes of Health.

Barry L. Jacobs, Ph.D., is currently a professor in the program of neuroscience at Princeton University. Professor Jacobs is author of *Serotonin Neurotransmission and Behavior* and *Hallucinogens: Neurochemical, Behavioral and Clinical Perspectives.* He has written many journal articles in the field of neuroscience and contributed numerous chapters to books on behavior and brain science. He has been a member of several panels of the National Institute of Mental Health.

Joann Ellison Rodgers, M.S. (Columbia), became Deputy Director of Public Affairs and Director of Media Relations for the Johns Hopkins Medical Institutions in Baltimore, Maryland, in 1984 after 18 years as an award-winning science journalist and widely read columnist for the Hearst newspapers.